D0615984

WITHDRAWN
FROM THE RECORDS OF THE
MID-CONTINENT PUBLIC LIBRARY

155.5 SA14
Sachs, Brad.
When no one understands

MID-CONTINENT PUBLIC LIBRARY
Blue Springs North Branch
850 N. Hunter Drive
Blue Springs, MO 64015 BN

WITHDRAWN
FROM THE RECORDS OF THE
MID-CONTINENT PUBLIC LIBRARY

WHEN
NO ONE
UNDERSTANDS

Also by Brad Sachs, PhD

The Good Enough Teen:
    Raising Adolescents with Love
    and Acceptance (Despite How
    Impossible They Can Be)

The Good Enough Child:
    How to Have an Imperfect Family
    and Be Perfectly Satisfied

Things Just Haven't Been the Same:
    Making the Transition
    from Marriage to Parenthood

WHEN NO ONE UNDERSTANDS

Letters to a Teenager
on Life, Loss,
and the
Hard Road
to Adulthood

BRAD SACHS, PhD

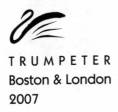

TRUMPETER
Boston & London
2007

MID-CONTINENT PUBLIC LIBRARY
Blue Springs North Branch
850 N. Hunter Drive
Blue Springs, MO 64015 **BN**

MID-CONTINENT PUBLIC LIBRARY - BTM

3 0003 00481795 1

Trumpeter Books
An imprint of Shambhala Publications, Inc.
Horticultural Hall
300 Massachusetts Avenue
Boston, Massachusetts 02115
www.shambhala.com

© *2007 by Brad Sachs*

*All rights reserved. No part of this book may be
reproduced in any form or by any means, electronic
or mechanical, including photocopying, recording,
or by any information storage and retrieval system,
without permission in writing from the publisher.*

9 8 7 6 5 4 3 2 1

First Edition

Printed in the United States of America

♾ *This edition is printed on acid-free paper that meets
the American National Standards Institute Z39.48 Standard.
Distributed in the United States by Random House, Inc.,
and in Canada by Random House of Canada Ltd*

Library of Congress Cataloging-in-Publication Data
Sachs, Brad, 1956–
*When no one understands: letters to a teenager on life, loss,
and the hard road to adulthood / Brad Sachs.—1st ed.*
p. cm.
ISBN: 978-1-59030-407-5 (pbk.: alk. paper)
1. Adolescent psychology. 2. Life. 3. Conduct of life. I. Title.
BF724.S23 2007
155.5—dc22
2006029792

—

This book is dedicated to:

"Amanda," and to all of my
other adolescent patients who
have been so forgiving of my
limitations, and who have
nonetheless taken the risk of
opening up to me the blossoming beauty
of their ambitious hearts

My three teenaged children,
Josh, Matt, and Jessica, who have
always kept me honest and humble
with their ever-so-gentle (yeah, right)
brand of mocking humor

And Karen, with love and gratitude
for all that we've created
and all that we share.

—

This is how he grows;
by being defeated decisively
by constantly greater things.

—Rainer Maria Rilke

—

Be kind, for everyone
you meet is fighting
a great battle.

—Philo of Alexandria

CONTENTS

NOTE TO THE READER

Names, as well as some identifying details, have been changed for the purpose of protecting Amanda's confidentiality as well as that of her friends and family.

Some of the letters to Amanda that follow are amalgams of text that was actually contained in two or more separate letters, and several contain a paragraph or two that were not in the original letters but have been inserted in order to smooth out the narrative flow and to help the reader understand the clinical material that I am responding to.

All of my original letters were written somewhat quickly, either at the end of a long day or between appointments, so in revisiting them and preparing them for publication, I have taken the liberty of doing some modest rewriting in order to clarify my thoughts for a general readership as well as to polish things up a bit stylistically.

Because the reader is not privy to the letters from Amanda that I am replying to, I have also decided to provide each letter with a title that is designed to act like a lens, helping to focus the reader's attention on the matters that I will be addressing.

Aside from these aforementioned changes, the letters that follow are, in their spirit and essence, the same letters that Amanda received, read, and responded to.

WHEN
NO ONE
UNDERSTANDS

PROLOGUE

One rainy November morning two taut and haggard parents arrived at my office with their sixteen-year-old daughter, Amanda, who had been discharged the day before from the hospital. Amanda had been in treatment for several years, and the week before, she had made a serious attempt at suicide: after swallowing dozens of pills, some prescribed, some over-the-counter, she had washed them all down with half a bottle of vodka.

Fortunately, one of her close friends knew something was up when she tried to instant message Amanda and encountered a morbid Away message. She then alertly called Amanda's mother when Amanda didn't answer her cell phone. Her mother discovered Amanda lying unconscious on the floor of her bedroom and called 911, and Amanda was transported by ambulance to the emergency room. Once medically stabilized, she was transferred to an inpatient psychiatric unit for three days and then released with the expectation that she participate in therapy. A colleague of mine who worked at the hospital provided the family with my name, and they called the next day to schedule their initial consultation.

Amanda, of course, like most of the adolescents I see, was coming under protest. Not only was it not her wish to be treated, but according to the previous therapists' notes, she seemed to assiduously resist *every* effort on *anyone's* part to promote change. Meanwhile, she had already been diagnosed with and treated for a wide range of mental illnesses—bipolar disorder, borderline personality disorder, dysthymic disorder, major depressive disorder, schizoaffective disorder, adjustment disorder, attention deficit disorder, and dissociative disorder.

At first Amanda was no different with me than she had been with any other well-meaning clinician. It appeared that she had taken a vow of snowy silence as she sat mutely before me, both when her parents were in the room and when she was alone with me, staring sullenly at the floor and slowly bobbing her head, as if to an invisible source of mesmeric music.

No stranger to situations of this sort—just like anyone else who works with adolescents in any capacity—and knowing that unconventional therapy, particularly with teens, is often the most effective therapy, I looked for other ways to bring about some contact, some growth, and some healing. Rather than attempt to cajole her into superficial, monosyllabic conversations, I took note from her clinical records that she was an avid reader and creative writer and decided to try to embark on a letter-writing relationship with her as a less invasive, more productive way of establishing a connection. For whichever of the indiscernible reasons that account for the mystery of human behavior, she decided to join me in this shared endeavor.

Recently, and somewhat fortuitously, Amanda attended a signing that I was doing at a local bookstore. Heartened to get an update and to see and hear how well she was doing as a young adult, I left the store in a reverie, marveling that for most of the first months of our treatment together, she had not said a single word to me during any of our sessions.

As I drove home from the book signing, it occurred to me that collecting and editing the letters that Amanda and I wrote to each other might provide a useful framework in which to share my thoughts about adolescent growth and development directly with teenagers as well as with parents of teenagers and with educators, clinicians, and other professionals who have committed themselves to working with young adults.

While I originally conceptualized this book as one that would include both sides of our correspondence, after sharing that version of the manuscript with selected colleagues, parents, and adolescents and soliciting their response, I came to the conclusion that limiting the text to *my* letters actually heightened my capacity to speak to the reader more intimately. So after much consideration I decided to cut the book in half and focus exclusively on the words that I struggled and dared, from my most empathic heart, to offer to Amanda, the words that became part of the rescue raft that carried and delivered her to safer psychic shores.

When No One Understands, then, is a synthesis of twenty-two of the more than fifty letters that I wrote to Amanda throughout the course of her therapy with me. While you will quickly observe that some of Amanda's difficulties and behaviors were more worrisome and extreme than those that you—or those whom you are rearing, teaching, or treating—might personally have encountered or displayed, you will gradually come to understand, as you read, that her journey serves to illuminate many of the most common and elemental conditions and contradictions inherent in every adolescent's life.

All teenagers, regardless of gender, generation, or background, must at some point engage in the universal, time-honored, and mythic struggle to navigate the bewildering, sometimes harrowing, pilgrimage from childhood into adulthood. While the specifics of that transformation will always vary from person to person and never match up precisely, there is always much more that we share and have in common than there is that is distinct and distinguishing.

So let me welcome you into the privacy of a therapeutic bond and share with you one-half of the conversation that Amanda and I created together. In learning more about how our relationship unfolded, you will find yourself better able to gaze into, perceive, comprehend, and honor your deepest fears, longings, sorrows, and dreams. And this will in turn nourish my sincerest hope and belief that the words on these pages will gently guide and fortify you as you set forth through the labyrinthine passages of adolescence that ultimately yield to the remarkable birth of your singular adult self.

1
—

An Invitation

—

Dear Amanda,

First of all, let's get something straight: you don't need to say a word to me when you are in my office. Talking is not the only way for two people to communicate with each other, to make contact with each other, to get to know each other. In fact, talk can sometimes interfere with understanding—that's one of the reasons that I'm writing to you, because I've found, over the years, that the written word often carries greater meaning and authenticity than the spoken word. Also, in looking over the clinical charts that the hospital sent over to me prior to our first session, I couldn't help noticing the consistent As and Bs in English that you have earned throughout your middle school and high school career, which no doubt means that you, too, already have a pretty good comfort level with reading and writing.

5

So here's the deal: you can be as silent as you want to be during our sessions, but I'd like to see if we can establish a conversation through writing to each other if we're not going to be talking to each other. I will write to you after each appointment with some of my thoughts and observations, and I'd like you to write back with yours—it's that simple.

My proposal may leave you wondering why we have to have any sessions at all if most of our dialogue is going to take place *outside* of those sessions. The answer is that I still want to get a look at you, even if you have nothing to say—people are always communicating, even if they're not saying anything—and also because I want to leave open the *possibility* for us to talk to each other, should you ever find that there is a reason for us to do so. Also, I'm still going to want to schedule meetings with you and your parents together so that I can hear what's on their minds and so that we can discuss any matters that might affect the family as a whole.

Don't misunderstand me—I am not asking you to be happy about this arrangement. In fact, I'm quite convinced that coming to appointments, and reading to and responding to a therapist's letters, are not high on any sixteen-year-old's list of fun activities. But I'm equally convinced that you are aware of the fact that your suicide attempt worried many people—your family, your friends, your teachers—so you're kind of stuck with me for now, at least until you can prove to everyone that you no longer need to be worried about. Since you're stuck with me, we might as well see if we can make the best of the situation and learn what we can from each other.

Once you've given this letter some consideration, let me know what you think, and then we'll take it from there.

Best regards,
Dr. Sachs

2

Why Bother?

———

Dear Amanda,

I appreciated your response to my letter, which I received yesterday. I was glad that you took the risk of being straight with me about your unwillingness to be "shrunk"; about your unhappy history with previous therapists who not only have not helped but have, at times, been downright insensitive; and about your lack of enthusiasm for any further psychological treatment. Frankly, I'd be a little skeptical if you had sounded chipper and optimistic at this point—after all, in looking over your chart, I counted up five different therapists whom you have already had to meet with over the years—so it's no wonder that you're not exactly turning cartwheels at the prospect of signing up with number six.

You wrote that you can already tell that I'm "just like all

the others," and that may, in fact, be true. I certainly don't know that I am going to be all that different from any of your other therapists. On the other hand, the fact that you were so clear about what made these clinicians ineffective—their desire to "change" you, their wish to "help" you, their belief that they "understood" you, their insistence that they "know what you're going through"—does at least give me the chance to avoid repeating some of their mistakes and perhaps try something new (or at least make some new mistakes).

If you want to know the truth, I'm not interested in changing you, I'm not sure you need or want my help, I don't understand you, and I really have no idea what you're going through. I do have to confess to being *interested* in you and curious about what has prompted you to consider ending your life when it's clear, based on my conversations with your family and other people who have gotten to know you, that you have a wide range of abilities and talents. But I don't think it's really my job to determine for you how you should live your life as a young adult and tell you what I think is best for you. Those conclusions and decisions are ones that *you* need to arrive at, and are always the result of a process of *self-discovery* rather than of being told what to do.

On the other hand, however, I would be lying if I didn't admit that I'd like you to stay alive long enough to make it through adolescence and see how things turn out—there are always some surprises along the way, and I wouldn't want you to miss out on any of them.

In any case, I was pleased that you made the time to write back and to express yourself so honestly, and I look forward to our unfolding conversation.

Best regards,
Dr. Sachs

3

—

Why Should I Go On?

—

Dear Amanda,

My letter to you today will mostly consist of my clumsy attempt to answer the question that you began and ended your most recent letter with: "Why should I go on?" It's a simple question, a profound question, in some ways the most elemental of all questions, the question that you have every right to ask, based on how much pain you have already had to encounter in your young life—and because of this, it's a question that deserves to be addressed.

The first answer that comes to mind, I must somewhat sheepishly admit, is "I don't know." That's not to suggest that you *shouldn't* go on, of course, that you should just toss in the towel and embark on one final suicidal mission. It's more of an acknowledgment of what you've already come to know, and what anybody with an open mind and a big heart comes to know—that life is hard, that life is a struggle, and that, as many have joked, no one gets out of it alive.

But when life is filled with despair, with anguish, with hopelessness, as yours currently is, it's fair to wonder what the point of continuing really is. To slog your way through this misery only to encounter more misery must seem futile indeed. I'm sure that plenty of people have tried to answer this question by enthusiastically telling you that "there's so much to live for," and you've probably concluded that they would have to be out of their minds to say this, completely incapable of understanding the depth of your suffering. Nonetheless, with all due respect for the state of mind that prompts you to pose this "life-and-death" query, here is my response:

The best reason to go on is because you cannot assume that your life is always going to feel the way it feels now. Adolescence, as you probably already understand, is an extremely complicated phase of life—the changes in one's mind, body, and soul are oceanic ones, and it's impossible to make it through without long, frequent, and difficult periods of confusion, upset, anxiety, and sorrow. On the other hand, adolescence is still a phase, and phases come and go. While you may feel absolutely whipsawed by your life right now, you cannot assume that the current state of affairs will remain constant—the nature of life is that it will always ebb and flow.

The main reason that you're struggling so much right now is that adolescence, surprising as this may sound, is a time of loss. This is something that many adults and teenagers don't understand. After all, adults are constantly telling teenagers, "This should be the best time of your life" or "Youth is wasted on the young" or "I wish I could go back in time and live those years over again." And of course teenagers, like you, are either left feeling bad about the fact that they're not enjoying their lives as much as they're "supposed to" or they find themselves wondering why any adult in their right mind would possibly want to return to such a tortured time of life.

When I talk about adolescence as a time of loss, the question you're probably asking is "What am I losing?" I suppose the best answer to that question is "your childhood," because we can never become a successful adult until we say good-bye to being a child. And that's exactly what is happening during adolescence—we're trying to find a resting place, a burial ground, for the child that we used to be, and trying to mourn her passing so that we can move on.

This is a task that is quite challenging because there's always sorrow when there's a death, and we lose a lot when we lose our childhood, even though we get a lot more in return. Perhaps the main thing we are losing is our precious treasure chest of childhood fantasies—fantasies that may have us convinced that we are the center of the universe, that we will always be taken care of, that everything will be better when we're older, that we can do anything we want, that we are invulnerable, that everything that is dear to us is easily within reach, that we will live forever. In releasing these fantasies we lay the groundwork for a real life—as a poet once said, "The best way to make dreams come true is to wake up"—but it can still be a lot easier to live in a fantasy world than in the real world.

I think one of the reasons that adolescents find themselves thinking a lot about death—even *stalking* death, as you appear to have been doing—is that at some level they're aware of and trying to confront the death of their childhood. The suicidal thoughts and attempts are not just efforts to relieve pain—to put yourself out of your misery—but are also a way to acknowledge that some part of us needs to die if some new part of us, our adult identity, is to be born. Of course, the irony of using suicide to deal with this issue is that it makes that very birth impossible—it's the "final solution," as they say, the solution that you can never return from. But it's important to consider the possibility that the *desire* to end your life is not something to be feared or vanquished but something to be welcomed and understood—just not something to be acted upon.

So rather than seeing your suicide attempt as some sort of symptom—a sign that you are emotionally disturbed or mentally ill or psychologically unbalanced—I would rather we think about it as part of your energetic effort to make the passage from childhood to adulthood. And maybe in subsequent meetings and letters we can discuss some other ways to make this passage that do not jeopardize the very life that is beginning to blossom.

With respect for your courage,
Dr. Sachs

4

What's Wrong with Me?

Dear Amanda,

I was impressed that you were able to give some thought and reflection to what I wrote to you in my last letter. Your willingness to look at your suicide attempt as something other than a psychiatric symptom, and to see it as rooted more in life than in death, shows great maturity and wisdom on your part. That it also led you to begin thinking about and questioning your "sanity or lack thereof" is, I think, a logical extension of our discussion.

You noted in your letter the many diagnostic categories in which you have been placed by your previous doctors and wondered which one, or ones, of those categories *I* would select for you. I'm not sure that I can answer that question because, while those categories can sometimes have value, they usually create more problems than they solve. In our efforts to try to make sense of the various kinds of distress and discomfort that people experience, I'm afraid that we have so narrowly defined what "normal" is that the slightest deviation from the norm is automatically diagnosed as a disease or disorder.

Take "depression," for example. We seem to live in a culture that holds forth the possibility of some kind of perpetual euphoria—we should always be happy, and if we're *not* happy, something must be wrong and that something must quickly be made right again. So if someone appears sad or depressed, that is automatically seen as a bad thing, a problem to be solved, a fracture to be fixed.

Somehow we seem to have lost track of the notion that there really are not positive emotions or negative emotions but that *all* emotions can teach us important things about ourselves if we allow them to. To me, a healthy person is defined as someone who can feel sad *as well as* happy, anxious *as well as* calm, insecure *as well as* self-confident. Legislating which emotions are okay and which are not makes it hard for us ever to feel comfortable in our own skin, since every emotion—even one that is not comfortably endured—yearns to be experienced and accepted.

This may sound a little strange, but I actually think it's important—even necessary—for us to go through periods of depression, because those may be the times when we are quieter and less active and thus more likely to be attentive to what is developing, emerging, and arising from inside us. If we were constantly "pumped up" we'd miss some of these very important aspects of ourselves, just as being constantly bombarded by loud music would cause us to miss the softer sounds of the world that deserve to be heard too.

I will grant you that depressive feelings can sometimes

get to be overwhelming and no longer serve a useful or important purpose—some researchers think this may be because of some unevenness in our neurochemistry—and it's appropriate at those times to assess and treat the condition so that one can live one's life fully. In fact, that is why you have been prescribed some of the medications that you have been taking, in an effort to try to even things out neurochemically and help you to reclaim some of your energy and vitality.

But remember that medicine is only a tool, and that there are many things that change our neurochemistry, as well. Activities such as exercising, writing, meditating, praying, eating right, and reading, to name a few, all affect our neurochemistry with a potency that equals—and often surpasses—that of a medication, and without any of the side effects that you have struggled with.

So I guess this is a roundabout way of saying that I'm not all that interested in what your diagnosis is, and unless I have to fill out a form that asks me to come up with one, I would just as soon see you as who you are, someone who is bigger than her symptoms, someone whose humanness cannot be confined by categories that may have some logic to them but cannot begin to contain and describe what makes you who you are.

Sorry if my response is a disappointing one, or not what you wanted to hear, but as you've given me the gift of your honesty I thought it was only fair to return the favor.

With appreciation for your patience,
Dr. Sachs

5

Why Is My Mom So Impossible?

Dear Amanda,

It was not difficult to get the impression from your most recent letter that you're feeling somewhat fed up with your parents. While this is not an uncommon state of affairs, particularly between a teenager and her mother and father, it deserves some thought and strategizing on our parts, as you're likely to remain at home with them for at least another couple of years, and I'm sure that everybody wants those years to be as livable as possible for all of you. After that, of course, when you're on your own, things tend to get a little easier.

One of your main jobs during adolescence is to become your own person, an individual who is unique, separate, and different from the family in which you have been raised. As part of that process, it's important that you examine your mother and father carefully, acknowledging their strengths and their weaknesses, coming to terms with their assets and their flaws. You will know you have done your job when you can accept your parents for who they are, despite their imperfections—after all, they were raised by imperfect parents, just like you, and just like all of us. So when I hear you complaining about your parents, I see it as a positive sign, a sign that you are beginning to think independently, a sign that you are on the road to becoming someone who can honor and embody what you find best about your parents and who can release and leave behind what you don't.

Your irritability with your mom is understandable—at a point in your life when you're wanting as much space and independence as possible, she's constantly monitoring and scrutinizing you, wanting to know how you're doing, asking you what you're up to, wondering what your plans are, what you're thinking, what you're feeling. It's not a surprise that you're feeling suffocated by her constant presence.

On the other hand, it's also not a surprise that she's being as present as she is. After all, a parent's biggest nightmare is something awful happening to her child, and let's face it, your recent suicide attempt was a pretty close call—it could have gone either way. So she may be desperately doing everything in her power, everything that she knows how to do, to try to prevent something tragic from happening to you again, and one of those things is knowing as much about you as she can.

Of course, you're probably thinking that she's making things worse by being so intrusive: "If she'd just back off and give me some space, I'd feel better—her being in my face all the time is *deadly*—it makes me want to *end* my life, not continue it," might be going through your head, and that's understandable. Whether you know it or not, however, you have some control over how involved with your life she is.

The thing is, parents *always* worry about their children, even when their children are no longer children. But if you can find a way to help her worry a little less, you might find that you create some of the breathing room that you hunger for at this point in your life. One way to help her worry less is to let her know some of the things that are going on in your life—information is the great antidote to parental worry.

Now, that doesn't mean that she has to, deserves to, or even *wants* to know every little detail about you. Nobody should or will know *everything* about you, and we all need to keep some parts of ourselves private and undetected—that's one of the ways we know we're our own person, by playing some cards close to the chest, by keeping some things to ourselves. But deciding to invite your mother into *certain* aspects of your life is likely to pay off in a big way—as she comes to understand you more, she's going to worry less, and when she's less worried, she's going to feel less need to be on top of you, and you'll feel freer, less like a hostage in your own home.

It's up to you, of course, to decide what you're going to disclose to her—it might be what's going on in school, it might be what's going on among your friends, it might be what's going on inside your very soul. But if you make it clear to her that you're not closing her out of your life en- tirely—if you become less of a cipher, less of a stranger, to her—you're going to have a more relaxed mom, and a more relaxed mom will mean a less stressed daughter.

At this point you might be thinking, "If I start to tell her what's going on in my life, she's just going to start prying and want to know more and more—if I give her an inch, she'll insist on taking a mile." That's a legitimate concern on your part, and your mom will have to learn to accept what you offer her and not insist on or demand more, if you're to keep the door open to her. But what I have seen, after having gotten to know a lot of parents over the years and being one myself, is that it's easier for us to back off when we're better informed about who we're backing off from. Being stingy with what you disclose to your mother is fine, but don't be *too* stingy or you'll wind up inviting the very controls that you're trying so hard to wriggle out of.

I am sure there are other things about your mother that are maddening, but why don't you start by giving some thought to my perspective, and then let me know how it goes.

With respect for your struggles,
Dr. Sachs

6

Why Is My Dad So Impossible?

Dear Amanda,

When you followed up my letter about your mom with a letter about your dad and surmised that "Dads are weird," I found myself thinking that I couldn't agree with you more. Your dad probably feels like a mystery to you now—in fact, just as much a mystery to you as you probably feel like to him.

What I know about your father, based on having spoken with him and with your mom, as well as from your letter, is that he was pretty involved in your life until just a couple of years ago, when he seemed to kind of disappear. Why that is, I'm not sure, but I *am* sure that this state of affairs must be a little confusing for you. Maybe if you had a better understanding of him, he'd seem less weird and a bit easier to deal with.

Psychologists, as you already know, often look to the past for clues about how a person behaves in the present. I know you are aware that your father had an older sister, Delia, who led a very tragic life. What I was told was that he and your Aunt Delia were quite close growing up, but once she started high school, her life started to take some sharp and dangerous turns. She became heavily involved with alcohol and drugs, she became a mother before she had even finished high school, she married unsuccessfully two times, and she was killed in a car accident that resulted from her drunk driving at the incredibly young age of twenty-four, when your father was in the middle of college.

I will tell you what I told your father—I don't believe that he's ever grieved for Delia, and I don't think he's ever come to terms with her death. Of course, it wasn't very easy to do this in your dad's family. Your mother told me that your father's parents, your paternal grandparents, still don't even mention Delia's name—it's as if they're so heartbroken about her death they can't even allow themselves to imagine that she was ever alive. So your dad probably had no place to go with all of his sadness about his sister—as a teenager, he had to stand by and watch helplessly as his big sister made poor choice after poor choice, gradually bringing her life to a sudden and premature end. Sometimes families come together around a painful loss and grow closer, warmer, tighter as a result. Your dad's family, for whatever reasons, could not do this. Nobody spoke, nobody cried, or if they *did* cry, they did so privately, and your dad had to bury his grief along with his sister.

What does this have to do with you and your relationship with him? Quite a bit, I believe. Because one of the perplexing things that parents do when they have a child is to search for things about their child that seem familiar to them, that remind them of someone they already know.

They notice that you sneeze like your grandmother or that you laugh like your uncle, that you sing like your father or that you sleep like your aunt.

Why do they do this? I guess the best way to explain it is that it helps them to do the hard work required of parenthood. Remember that when you're born, you're a kind of stranger to your parents—they haven't met you before, but they're supposed to devote all of this time and energy to taking care of you. That's going to be a lot easier to justify if you seem a little more familiar to them—after all, who wants to wake up in the middle of the night to feed and change the diaper of someone who doesn't appear to have any connection with them? So they instantly apply themselves to figuring out who you remind them of so that you seem a little less strange, a little more recognizable. This process happens not only when parents have a child by birth but also with adoptive parents, stepparents, and foster parents.

Sometimes this creates problems, however, particularly if the person you remind them of is someone whom they have a complicated relationship with. And that, I believe, is what's going on with your dad right now. Without meaning to, simply by being a female teenager, you are reminding him of his sister—and his sister, without ever meaning to, caused your father great pain. He has mostly dealt with that pain by trying to avoid it, and I think that may be why he's avoiding *you*. After all, as you said in your letter, the two of you used to "do stuff together—go for bike rides, play cards, walk the dog"—and now you don't even talk. So it's kind of like what happened between him and Delia—years of closeness, and then all of a sudden a lot of distance.

I'm not excusing your dad's behavior, just trying to explain it. Because I think that when we can understand someone's behavior, we are better able to manage our response to it. Something that's important to remember in all of this is that it really isn't your fault that your dad has pulled away from you. After all, there's not a whole lot you can do about the fact that you remind him of his sister—that was going to happen anyway, and *has* been happening for years. On the other hand, how close you have already come to an early death through your suicide attempt is probably reinforcing for your dad the ways in which you remind him of Aunt Delia, making it that much harder for him to get past his grief and be a better dad. "Why get close to Amanda when she's just going to abandon me, like Delia did?" would be, you'd have to admit, a logical question for him to ask himself, even subconsciously.

One thing I've asked your father to do already is to give some more thought to his relationship with his sister and to try to find some ways to reconnect with her, even though she's dead. Just because she's no longer alive doesn't mean that he can't remember her fondly, that he can't recall the closeness that didn't last as long as they had wanted it to but was important and meaningful just the same for how long it did last. I have learned over the years that while death signals the end of *life,* it doesn't have to signal the end of *love,* or the end of a relationship with the loved one who has passed on. Perhaps if he can reopen his heart to his love for his sister, he'll be better able to reopen his heart to his love for you and show you that love in some of the ways that he used to, and in new ways as well.

What can you do to help this along? One suggestion is to try to learn more about Aunt Delia, because I believe that she's been an important person in your life even though she died years before you were born. Ask your father if he might tell you more about her. See if he's got any pictures of her. If you're comfortable, ask him if he'd go with you to see where she's buried. These might seem like odd or creepy things to do, but in a funny way, bringing your aunt "back to life" by talking about and remembering her might help *you* come back to life, too, a life that might flourish in all the ways that Aunt Delia's could have but never did.

With understanding,
Dr. Sachs

7

How Do I Live with a Broken Heart?

Dear Amanda,

While I was impressed that you began talking to me directly during our last session together, I could see how difficult it was for you to do so and want to remind you that our letters to each other can and will continue as long as we'd like them to—trying out or exploring one form of communication doesn't eliminate the importance of any others.

In the meantime, I did want to convey to you some of my responses to what you were telling me, and writing to me, regarding the breakup with your boyfriend, a breakup that you thought might have contributed to your feeling hopeless enough to try to end your life.

Intimate relationships are wondrous but enormously complicated experiences. It sounded to me like your relationship with Peter was one that had great depth to it, a connection that was much more than a typical teen romance. When two bright, sensitive individuals are exclusively dating for almost eight months and sharing as much as the two of you shared with each other, a very significant bond is built. And it's a tremendous accomplishment to experience and cultivate that bond, particularly at your age.

I know from your letter that you feel that Peter was the one who ended things, who dumped you, and that that led to very hurt and very angry feelings. But I could also sense, as you described the arc of your relationship with each other, that things were starting to fray before that—you mentioned that you had been getting a little tired of his calling and texting you every night, of his getting upset if you wanted to spend time with your friends on the weekends, of his feeling threatened if you were talking to or instant messaging other guys.

What was going through my mind as I read was that you were the one who was actually fed up with the relationship before he was, but that perhaps you weren't sure that he was strong enough to tolerate being without you, so you hung in there with him until he could be the one to end it so you wouldn't have to feel guilty about hurting him. Of course, it's unlikely you were thinking this consciously—we psychologists have this annoying habit of looking into the unconscious, the part of our mind that directs a lot of our thoughts, feelings, and behaviors without our even being aware of it. But even though it may not have been a conscious decision on your part, I still think there's a strong possibility that your desire to protect Peter from hurt feelings was what led you to *allow* him to make the final decision to break up.

If you are now wondering, "Well, if *I* was the one who

wanted to end things more than *him,* then why did I get so bummed out when it actually happened?" then you're doing exactly what you should be doing, which is trying to learn as much as you can about yourself, particularly from events that are painful ones. And one plausible answer would be that you weren't so much bummed out about the fact that things were over (even though there's always some sadness when a close relationship comes to the end of its road) as about the fact that you had sacrificed yourself to make things easier on him.

Relationships always require sacrifices, but some sacrifices are better to make than others. And whenever we make sacrifices, we feel some anger about having to give up some part of ourselves—our power, our autonomy, our voice. I think you were upset about the end of your relationship with Peter not so much because it ended, or because he ended it, as because you permitted him to do to *you* what you had wanted to do to *him*—you set it up so that he would be the wounder and you would be the wounded.

I am not saying this to criticize you or to make you feel bad, Amanda. On the contrary, as I said, in my estimation it's a remarkable achievement to keep a relationship going as long as the two of you did. But it does appear that somewhere along the line you made the decision—conscious or unconscious—to take better care of Peter than of yourself, and I think that's why you were left with so much hurt and anger.

Your job is not to feel bad about this or regret it—as someone once told me, the three responses to a mistake should be admitting it, not repeating it, and learning from it. I would rather you give some thought to whether my take on your relationship has some relevance, to see how it felt to make the decision that you made, and to look at your other relationships to see if you tend to make similar, or different, sacrifices and how it feels to do so.

Either way, I want you to remember that the pain that you were feeling when things ended with Peter is pain that can help you to grow, that can ready you for your next relationship, and that can deepen you and your capacity to give and receive love.

With admiration for your courage,
Dr. Sachs

8

—

Why Do I Get High?

—

DEAR AMANDA,

I think it's safe to say that yesterday's session was not an easy one for you or your parents. They, as you know, are convinced that you came home drunk from a party this past weekend—they saw you stagger, they heard you slur words, they know you were up vomiting in the shower most of the night. You didn't say anything as they were describing things to me during the session, and as I've told you, it's your right not to—although I'm assuming, should you have felt that they were off base, that you would have spoken up to the contrary.

I am going to assume that, as an intelligent sixteen-year-old, you know the basics about drug and alcohol use, so I'm not going to waste my time or yours with a lecture—you've most likely had plenty of that already. I'm also not interested in getting you to admit that you were "bad" or that you "showed poor judgment," whether you feel this way or not. What I am interested in is *your* knowing more about the appeal of intoxicating substances—in other words, the answers to questions like what you enjoy about them, when you're tempted by them, how you decide whether or not to use them, and how much of them to use when you do.

It's really impossible for teenagers not to have some curiosity about drugs and alcohol—after all, we live in a very drug-drenched culture. These days there are pills for just about anything—headaches, stomachaches, anxiety, depression, shyness, inattentiveness, hyperactivity, fatigue, sleeplessness, obsessions and compulsions, sexual problems—the list goes on and on. Meanwhile, we're all constantly bombarded by advertisements for beer, wine, and hard liquor. And then there are the street drugs—pot, cocaine, heroin, assorted pills—that just about every high school student is exposed to in one form or another. So who wouldn't find themselves tempted to at least try one or more of these chemicals, legally or illegally?

But maybe we could begin to discuss this complicated matter in a thoughtful manner. One place to start would be for you to let me know more about the role that drugs and alcohol currently play in your life. For now, I would be willing to keep this information confidential, just between you and me, and would promise not to share it with your parents or anyone else. However, you would have to understand that if at any point I decide that there's something very worrisome about your use of drugs and alcohol, I would encourage you to talk to your parents about this and/or fill them in myself—although I wouldn't do so without letting you know ahead of time that I was going to.

Remember, Amanda, I'm not looking to change you or get you in trouble, and I'm not going to think any less of you based on what you choose to confide in me—you are still who you are, no matter what you do. But I do think that decisions about substance use are very important and difficult ones to make, and it's often valuable to get the perspective of an adult in addition to the perspective of your friends so that you can make the best decision possible.

On the other hand, should you decide that you *don't* want to fill me in with any more detail on this matter, I will respect your decision, and we'll just put that issue to the side for now.

Think about it, and, as always, I'll await your response.

Appreciatively,
Dr. Sachs

9
—

Am I Hooked?

—

Dear Amanda,

I received your letter, and it was good to know that you felt that a more in-depth discussion of drug and alcohol use would be worthwhile—I think that shows a lot of maturity on your part. I also appreciated your trust in me, and just so you know, based on what you shared, I am not feeling the need to broach this subject with your parents at this time— as I said, I'll let you know if we get to that point.

You mentioned that you've been smoking pot "often" for almost a year now, that you binge drink now and then, and that you've "messed with some other things, like Ecstasy and acid," but haven't used them regularly, and that you'll never touch tobacco because "it's gross."

What I was particularly impressed by in your letter was

your awareness of what drugs do for you—for example, you said that when you smoke pot, you feel more relaxed, you laugh more easily, and you appreciate music more fully. Drugs like marijuana would not be as popular as they are unless there were something appealing about them, and you have clearly identified some of the most commonly sought-after effects of using this substance.

While you have been reassuring yourself that it's okay to smoke on a daily basis because it's not "addictive," I do want you to give some further consideration to this issue. Individuals who consistently smoke pot may not go through physical withdrawal when they do decide to give it up, but there is still a difficult emotional withdrawal that has to be dealt with. You're certainly in the habit of smoking pot right now, and as you know, there are some risks associated with this, risks that, to avoid sounding repetitive, I'll assume you're aware of (although we can discuss these, too, at some point if you'd like).

And sometimes when we use a drug regularly for emotional reasons, such as to feel better, it actually diminishes our body's capacity to feel better on its own, which means that we become more and more dependent on the drug to do what we'd really like to be able to do independently (since the drug may not always be available to us).

Of course, the best way to tell whether you're addicted to a substance is to see if you can do without it and what happens to you when you're doing without it. Just for curiosity's sake, you might try an experiment in which you give up pot for a week and simply assess how you feel—the point being to observe yourself as a way of gaining a better understanding of what role it plays in your life. Maybe you could jot down some notes or keep a journal for those few days and, if you're comfortable, share these with me as well.

In any case, as I said in my previous letter, what you had

to say about your use of drugs and alcohol doesn't change the way I think about you—you're still Amanda, and you're still a wonderful, evolving young woman with many fine attributes and qualities. I was grateful that you invited me into this part of your life so that we have the chance to explore it together.

By the way, before I finish up, I couldn't help noticing some scratch marks on your arm that weren't there the last time you were in—what happened?

Just wondering,
Dr. Sachs

10

Why Must I Be Who Everyone Else Wants Me to Be?

—

Dear Amanda,

I wanted to get back to you about something from yesterday's session, your parents' sense that you have a great deal of artistic ability but that you rarely allow others to see it. They told me that while you'll spend much time sketching and drawing in your room, and numerous teachers over the years have told you that you're quite gifted, you won't take any art classes at school or at the local community center, and you refuse to put together a portfolio of your best work and consider entering competitions. This bothers them and makes them wonder why you don't believe in yourself.

One lesson I've learned from having gotten to know many creative individuals over the years is that creativity is a very precious possession, something that is unique and quite dear to us. That is why it's not unusual for artistically minded individuals to at times try to protect that creativity by keeping it to themselves, to tend and nurture it privately without exposing it to public scrutiny. It's as if once they bring it out into the world for others to see and experience, it's no longer theirs.

While I think it's marvelous that you have the capacity to express yourself artistically, as well as through writing, I also think that there's a certain intuitive wisdom in your keeping your work to yourself for now. I believe there's entirely too much emphasis on getting attention and acclaim in our culture, to win awards and contests and competitions in every range of endeavor. All this tends to do is prevent individuals from finding their own voice and their own ability, because they quickly become too preoccupied with what others think of their art and not focused enough on the art itself.

By doing what you're doing, you will give your artistry a chance to blossom on its own, at its own pace, in its own way. And that's the only way that it can truly become yours, that it can gratify and satisfy you and convey what you want it to convey. For now, I believe that you can trust that you will know when you're ready to invite the external world to share your creative accomplishments and that, until that time, you're entitled to keep it within yourself. I wish that more creative individuals, both adolescent and adult, understood this....

In the meantime, should you ever want to bring any creative pieces to one of our sessions, I'd be honored to take a look, although I would want to do so not to critique them but simply to become acquainted with another, deeply important part of you. So think about whether you might like to do that at some point—either way is okay with me.

Best regards,
Dr. Sachs

P.S. I appreciated your getting back to me about how the scratches on your arm came about, but something about your explanation—scraping it when you were reaching into your locker at school for some books—didn't quite ring true. If I'm off base here, just let me know, and please accept my apology for not having believed you. If there's more to the story, though, feel free to let me know that as well, even if you don't feel like getting into the *whole* story. You're certainly not expected or obligated to tell me everything that goes on in your life, but I'd just like to know whether my concern is warranted.

11

Why Am I Hurting Myself?

—

DEAR AMANDA,

I harbor a great deal of respect for you for detailing with greater truth how the scratches on your arm arose. Your acknowledging that you've been cutting yourself and that there are also cuts on your thighs and stomach that nobody else has yet seen, which I wouldn't have known about had you not told me, took a lot of courage on your part.

I also heard very clearly your concern that if you told me that you were cutting yourself, I would instantly arrange for you to be hospitalized again, something that you didn't want to happen.

I want to be very clear with you about this matter of hospitalization, just so there isn't any confusion—if I have any indication that you are considering ending your life, I won't hesitate to have you hospitalized so that you can be carefully supervised until the urge passes. On the other hand, I would strongly prefer that you live your life outside the hospital (as, I suspect, you would too), and I don't think that behaviors such as cutting yourself or smoking pot automatically dictate that you be treated as an inpatient.

So, for now, as long as we can establish a useful dialogue about your cutting, you needn't worry that you're going to automatically wind up in a psychiatric ward as a result of your candor.

On to the matter at hand . . . I must confess that there's something about self-cutting that has always intrigued me. The reason is that in many traditional cultures, and at many other times in human history, scarring oneself is not seen as symptomatic or problematic but is actually understood as a common ritual signifying that the transformation from childhood to adulthood is taking place. The scratch or cut or slice seems to function as a symbolic "dividing line" that separates who we were from who we are becoming. And the resultant scar is a constant and visible reminder that we have successfully navigated an important rite of passage, that we have "made it through" and can celebrate the acquisition of a new, more mature identity.

So, because all rites of passage involve a good amount of struggle, the etches on our skin wind up representing the etches on our soul that result from the struggle to shed our childhood and take on the mantle of young adulthood.

The problem in our culture, as I see it, is not that teens cut but that we, as a society, haven't created the meaningful rituals that would adequately help teens to feel that they've actually made the transition from child to adult. Sure, adolescents are eventually allowed to drive, drink, vote, apply to and attend college, and volunteer for the armed services, but those events occur much more toward the middle and end of adolescence than at the beginning. So, in a way, when I see teens cutting themselves, I'm fascinated because I have the sense that they are instinctively turning to a universal method of ritualizing the journey from being a child to being an adult, and they are doing so because our society, as a whole, isn't providing them with healthy, clearly defined customs that conduct them into and officially inaugurate young adulthood.

You may feel some embarrassment or shame about your cutting—and I suspect you do because you were hesitant to acknowledge it when I first asked about the scratches on your arm—but rather than feel embarrassed and ashamed, I believe it would be more productive to see the cutting as a way to demonstrate to yourself and others that you are evolving into a young woman and saying your good-bye to girlhood. The fact that you view the world so artistically would make it even more likely that you would want to find some visually riveting way to reinforce and display your transfiguration (in thinking back to my previous letter to you, perhaps you are, indeed, finding a way to share your artistic sense with the world, with your body as the "canvas" on display).

Now, this is not to say that your slicing yourself is without risks. There are physical dangers associated with this, such as accidentally slicing a vein or artery or infecting yourself if you're using an unsterilized implement. And there are social dangers, too—many people will be upset when they see these scratches and react in ways that you might not like, concluding that you are sick or abnormal, that something is drastically wrong with you, when, in reality, so much is right.

But the *urge* to carve or slash yourself is not, in itself, something that is worrisome or unhealthy. On the contrary, to me it speaks of a wholesome desire to usher yourself forward and to declare, to yourself and others, your ripening, your readiness to take on the responsibilities and privileges that come with age and maturity.

So I guess one thing you might want to think about is how to artistically portray the profound changes that you are in the midst of in a way that doesn't have any physical or social risk attached to it. Perhaps you could draw on your body with lipstick or henna or some other medium as a way of depicting your evolution. Perhaps you could create a painting or sculpture that might evoke and embody the experience of releasing yourself from one identity as you prepare to take on a new one. If you are not familiar with Tchaikovsky's ballet *Swan Lake,* you might want to go see a stage version of it or get hold of the DVD, as it is a remarkable evocation, through dance and music, of the painful but ultimately redemptive beauty associated with metamorphosis.

In any case, I'll be interested in seeing what you come up with, Amanda, and wanted to commend you again for your willingness to disclose to me something that you felt needed to be kept secret but that, to my way of thinking, is really just further evidence of your transformation.

With high regard for your fearlessness,
Dr. Sachs

12

—

How *Dare* You

—

DEAR AMANDA,

I can tell from your last letter that you are very angry with me, and you certainly don't have to explain why. When your parents asked me whether they should begin drug testing you because of their concerns and suspicions, and I agreed that they should, I didn't have any difficulty imagining that you would be furious.

You complained to me that the drug testing was intrusive, which it is, that it violates your privacy, which it does, and that it suggests that I don't trust you, which is true, insofar as I don't think that you are always completely honest with your parents or me (or even, perhaps, with yourself) regarding whether and when you get high and how much you feel the need to.

Without expecting you to relinquish your anger at me, however, I do want to very briefly explain to you the rationale behind my suggestion. Both you and your parents have grown weary of the ongoing and ultimately pointless debates regarding whether you are smoking pot. Your mom and dad worry every time your behavior is odd or your eyes are red or your mood is testy or you dash into the house and go right up to your room without checking in and saying hi. So, of course, when they're worried they ask you if you've gotten high, and you always say no, and they don't believe you, and you get frustrated with them, and they get aggravated with you, and the cycle goes on and on and on.

The advantage of the drug testing is that these unpleasant, unproductive interrogations can be put to rest. If the test shows up positive, your parents will know that you've been smoking and they will be able to address that matter at home with you and in sessions with me. If the test shows up negative, you no longer have to explain or defend yourself and your parents will more comfortably back off.

You probably know that many adults, such as professional athletes, actually request regular drug testing for just this reason, so that if there are any noticeable changes in their performance, for better or worse, it cannot be attributed to drug use and result in finger-pointing and unjust, inaccurate accusations.

So when I concurred with the idea of drug testing, it wasn't with the idea of making your life harder but, in fact, to make everybody's life easier.

That having been said, let me move on to the more important part of this letter, which has to do with what it's like for you to be so mad at me and to feel so betrayed.

You wrote, at the end of your letter, that having read all that you said, I probably wouldn't want to hear from you, see you, work with you, or write to you ever again. In reality,

Amanda, nothing could be further from the truth. The fact that you cared enough about the relationship that we have been building with each other to express your outrage, rather than just bottle it up and keep it to yourself or express it only to others but not to me, leads me to feel even more impressed with how much you've grown in the time we've gotten to know each other.

One of the oldest psychological definitions of depression is anger that is turned inward rather than outward—in other words, anger that is misdirected toward oneself rather than toward the individual(s) who might be more deserving of it. So, from my vantage point, your capacity to be angry with me and to drive it so forcefully in my direction means that you're going to be less prone to depression, which is a good thing. In fact, you might want to observe your mood over the course of the next few days and see if you notice any movements, even subtle ones, toward feeling less depressed.

In addition, I don't think it's really possible to have a meaningful relationship without some anger showing up at one point or another. Obviously we don't want it to be the predominant emotion that we share with another person, but I think that we make a big mistake when we operate under the assumption that we can have an important inter-personal connection without either party feeling angry now and then.

So, as far as I'm concerned, I've got plenty of room for you to be mad at me, and while I hope that you come to un-derstand that my support of drug testing was not with the intention of making things worse for you but, ultimately, to make things better, I also hope that you won't ever feel that being mad at me means that I won't want to hear from you or that I'll stop caring about you or that our relationship has to come to an end.

You've taken an important step by voicing your protest to me so frankly and straightforwardly, Amanda. I hope that it's the first of many times that you do so, not only with me but with others, and that you begin to see the far-reaching value of doing so.

With a continued commitment to staying connected,
Dr. Sachs

13

Why Am I So Lonely?

Dear Amanda,

You mentioned in your last letter the "terrible, crushing loneliness" that you feel these days, a loneliness that seems to be worse than it has ever been before. This may seem a little strange, but I want to take some time to tell you why I believe your being lonely is actually a good sign and why it's very important that you experience it right now.

As we have discussed before, you are at a phase in your life during which it's necessary for you to begin separating yourself from others—from your parents, from some of your friends, even, to some extent, from yourself and who you used to be. Whenever we begin the process of separating from someone or something important, we are prone to feeling lonely.

That's why little children will sometimes want to take a teddy bear or a doll with them to bed or to their babysitter's house or their preschool—these objects help them to deal with the intense loneliness they feel when they are experiencing their first separations from their parents, whom they have been used to spending all of their time with.

The separation that you are in the midst of right now, although different in many ways, is still no less profound than that of the toddler who feels frightened and overwhelmed when she is without the people who have been providing her with a sense of safety and security. You are realizing that you can no longer count on other people to take care of you in the way that they used to and that you need to begin taking care of yourself.

When this reality begins to emerge—and that's what I believe is happening for you right now—it's as if we were standing on the edge of a great, yawning abyss, one that has been emptied of everything but our own fears, our own anxieties, our own longings. It is difficult to imagine experiencing anything but a "terrible, crushing loneliness" when we stand on the edge of that abyss and can hear only the forlorn echo of our own desolate aloneness.

But that same loneliness, terrifying and immense as it may be, is telling us something essential. It is declaring that we are ready to leave our childhood behind, that we have started to release ourselves from the connections that have served a purpose until now but that have been outgrown and have actually begun to hinder us and hold us back.

Believe it or not, it is impossible to travel successfully and completely from childhood into adulthood without spending a serious amount of time contemplating loneliness, because the loneliness that seems to loom so ominously is actually nothing more than our mature self, the adult soul that has opened up and is welcoming us, inviting us to enter and inhabit it.

You wondered, in your letter, if your loneliness had to do with not being "attractive," with not having a "good personality," with being a "misfit." But I don't think it has anything to do with any of that. After all, you've also said that you've had close friends over the years, and while I expect you'll fight me on this one, most of the individuals I've spoken to who know you well, such as family members and teachers, say that you display much warmth and a quiet charm.

So, rather than find a way to blame yourself for your loneliness (and I must say, you've developed quite an advanced capacity for self-blame over the years; that's something we may want to examine at some point), I think it would be better to find a way to shake hands with your loneliness and become better acquainted with it. It's not going to be a permanent state and is, to my way of thinking, just further evidence that you are evolving.

One other thing that I want to remind you of that's working in your favor is that highly creative individuals such as you often find themselves to be outcasts as teenagers. The reason for this is that one of the easiest and safest ways to make it through adolescence is to conform, to become as much like everyone else as possible. While this works for some students, it works against someone who, like you, takes such justifiable pride in her uniqueness and out-of-the-ordinariness.

However, should you proceed with your stated plans to go to college or an art institute, you will eventually find yourself with many like-minded peers who also value originality over conventionality, imagination over compliance.

That, along with your gradually becoming more comfortable occupying your new, adult identity, will help to take the edge off the loneliness and keep it from feeling so oppressive.

Despite my sense that this will become less of a problem over time, though, I do sincerely hope that you never lose the capacity to feel lonely, because it is when we are lonely that we are not only most true to who we are but also most open to the possibility of who we may become. We don't live in a culture that values aloneness, that creates room for solitude, so sometimes we have to seek it for ourselves.

And one more thing—don't forget that writing to me about being lonely will help you make sense of your loneliness. I'm very glad that you were able to step out of yourself long enough to do so.

Your partner in aloneness . . .
Dr. Sachs

14

Why Does
My Brother Have
to Be So Perfect?

Dear Amanda,

In this afternoon's letter, I wanted to get back to what came up in our most recent session. When I was first getting to know you, you once described your older brother, Craig, as the "crown prince" of the family, and, indeed, he does seem to be enthroned. Your parents seem absolutely enamored with him and all that he does—he gets good grades in school, he's a talented athlete, he's good-looking and quite popular. They seem to have no complaints about him whatsoever, and whenever I've asked how he's doing, they are quick to fill me in on his many achievements and accomplishments. It's as if he were perfect in their eyes and can simply do no wrong.

In a recent letter, you wrote about how unfair things

seem to be at home, how there has been a "double standard" over the years, with Craig always getting the acclaim, the credit, and the benefit of the doubt, while you always receive the blame, the criticism, and the short end of the stick.

I find this arrangement particularly interesting based on the events of this past weekend that your parents filled me in on, in which (as you well know) Craig hosted a party for friends at your house while you and your parents were away visiting your grandparents, a party that got out of hand and led to several alcohol citations, including one that was handed out to your supposedly spotless and virtuous brother.

What struck me about your parents' account of the story fits in with your perception that there is a double standard in your home—while they were upset with Craig's lack of judgment, they didn't seem particularly angry with him, nor had they imposed any kind of consequence on him for having so flagrantly broken the rules (although that may change after the telephone discussion they had with me the other night). Apparently, to their way of thinking, the alcohol citation that he received and whatever legal ramifications result from this are "enough punishment" for him.

You mentioned, in one of your first letters to me, that Craig does a lot of drinking, more than your parents know about or, better, more than they perhaps *want* to know about. You've also wondered, on numerous occasions, why you seem to have always had the tendency to "screw up," particularly when things are finally starting to turn around for you.

By way of explanation, I want to propose something to you that may not make a lot of sense at first but that I want you to mull over anyway.

Do you remember back when we were discussing your breakup with Peter and I proposed that you had sacrificed yourself for him? I believe that for a very long time you have been assigned, and have obediently accepted, the role of sacrificing yourself for Craig, protecting him and keeping him elevated and enshrined on the pedestal that your parents have so lovingly created for him.

And I believe that one of the ways in which you fulfill that role is to continue to create enough difficulties that Craig always looks very good in comparison with you, and such that your parents' attention is always diverted away from his problems and onto yours.

Now, once again, I am not saying that you are necessarily conscious of playing this role—in fact, one of the reasons I am bringing this out is because I want to make you more aware of motivations that seem to lie outside of your awareness. After all, as we've already seen, when we understand the basis for our behavior, invisible as it may have been, it becomes that much easier to change that behavior. But I want you to think about this possibility nonetheless, because I am convinced it would explain a lot of what goes on.

To make my point a little clearer, let me give you some background. In an earlier letter to you, I suggested that one of the reasons that your father might be having difficulty staying connected with you was that you reminded him of his younger, self-destructive sister, Delia. Another piece of your family history that your parents have told me about, which you already know, is that the first two times that your mother became pregnant, she experienced miscarriages.

Repeated miscarriages, as you can well imagine, fill a couple with unimaginable pain. Your parents handled this to the best of their ability and naturally went on to try to start a family again, which they were obviously successful in doing.

But one of the things that sometimes happens after a loss of the sort that your parents experienced is that they exalt the baby who finally comes to term, the one who survives—in this case, Craig. They feel *so* grateful, *so* blessed, and *so* happy to have a healthy child that that child can "do no wrong."

Of course, no child is perfect, even the one who restores parents' faith after such misfortune. So a mother and father will have to work very hard to ignore all the flaws and problems that the anointed child displays in order to keep him bathed in the pure light of perfection and keep them safe from the unbearably painful memories of their lost children.

Something that can help this process along is to have a second child, because this child can then become the container of all the flaws and defects and problems that they don't want to imagine that the first child has. With a "bad child" now in the picture, it is that much easier for the parents to take pride in the "good child."

In a way, it's like what happens in the Bible, when a single goat is designated as the "scapegoat" and the entire community symbolically loads the scapegoat with all of their collective sins and then sends the goat off into the wilderness so that they can be ritualistically cleansed of their transgressions. The "bad child" is the family scapegoat, serving the important purpose of taking on and carrying off every other family member's negative load so that they are all left free, unblemished, and clear.

The problem, of course, is that in most cases nobody is aware of this complicated process taking place. The parents truly believe that one child is better than the other and, of course, get into the habit of treating that child better, which just reinforces the whole imbalance, because it's much easier to be good if you're treated like you're all good or, conversely, to be bad if you're treated like you're all bad.

Just as important, the children themselves may come to believe that one child is better than the other. The first child will literally think that he can "do no wrong," as if this were a fact, and the second child will literally think that she can "do no right," as if this were just as true.

Siblings often get locked into their respective roles, and this, I think, is what has happened in your family. Without knowing it, you've accepted the family's designation of you as the family scapegoat, the scapegoat that keeps them from owning or accepting responsibility for problems or difficulties that each of them has, and you have become wedded to the belief that your ultimate value is in creating problems and difficulties so that your peerless, impeccable brother can continue to dazzle and shine.

So you complain to me that your parents refuse to notice your brother's drinking problem, but you simultaneously create so many other problems that they have no reason to look very carefully at his behavior or take it very seriously when he crosses the line, even dangerously, as he did last week.

That is why I want you to think about why you make it so easy for your brother to be the "perfect son," why you work so conscientiously to be the "imperfect daughter," and whether it's such a good idea for you to continue sacrificing yourself to preserve Craig's reign as the "crown prince." Every family member will at times be a little bit of a scapegoat, but more severe problems occur when one individual becomes the only scapegoat, and I suspect that is what has happened in your family.

One thing you will have to be prepared for is that if you do decide to give up the scapegoat role and allow yourself to move forward, the family's equilibrium is going to change. Your parents may begin to become more concerned about Craig's imperfections, or he may try to find ways to push you back down into the scapegoat role to protect and preserve his royalty, a position he's been getting a lot out of.

Give this some thought, and let's see what develops as you experiment with doing things a little differently.

As always, thanks for tolerating some of my "illogical" hypotheses and speculations—I'd understand if you thought I was a little nuts, but I hope you'll bear with me nonetheless.

Best regards,
Dr. Sachs

15
—

Am I Ready to Have Sex?

—

Dear Amanda,

You are going to be either relieved or upset by the topic of this letter—probably some combination of both—but I'm hoping that, as we've known each other for some time now, you'll receive it in the spirit in which it was written.

In my last meeting with your parents, which you did not attend because you were sick, your mom told me that you had asked her to arrange for you to get birth control pills and she wasn't sure what to do or how to respond. Having spoken to them about this matter, I also wanted to share with you some of my thoughts in the hopes that I can assist you and your parents in making the best decision possible.

First of all, for several different reasons I am pleased to hear that you made this request. One, it suggests that your relationship with Dante, whom I understand you've been seeing for a few months now, is growing closer. Two, it shows that you are thinking ahead to what kind of sexual intimacy the two of you would like to share and that you wish to prevent an unwanted pregnancy by using safe and available contraception. Three, it demonstrates a desire on your part to talk to your mother about an important personal matter, which is an indication that you're feeling a little more trusting of her.

So, for all of these reasons, it's promising, from my perspective, to hear that this issue is on the table for you, and I certainly wish that more teenagers were willing to talk to adults about decisions that are this significant rather than feeling that they have to make complicated choices all by themselves or only with the input of their friends. Since I'm one of those adults, I hope you'll tolerate my throwing in my two cents.

Sexual pleasure is one of the most special and profound of all pleasures, if for no other reason than that it is at its best when experienced in the context of a relationship with another person. In fact, I've always felt a little frustrated by some of the sex education that is offered to children and teens, because while there is an understandable and important emphasis on being healthy and responsible—which you're clearly responding to by looking into effective birth control—there is little emphasis on how enjoyable sexual intimacy can and should be.

So I believe that our society makes it quite difficult for young men and women such as you and Dante to make good decisions about what kind of sexual activity to engage in. On the one hand, we constantly bombard you with images in magazines, movies, television shows, and advertisements and on the Internet that emphasize the "joy of sex" and make it all seem so effortless, carefree, casual, and spontaneous. At the same time, you're constantly warned—at times in terrifying ways—about the many risks of sexual interest and activity, such as pregnancy, STDs, rape, and the potential for emotional hurt and humiliation.

I would also have to say that despite some positive cultural changes over the last few decades as a result of feminism, sexual decision making for girls remains particularly complicated. I still observe a double standard, both from parents and from teens, suggesting that girls are not and should not be all that interested in sex, and if they are, they must be "whores" or "sluts" (guys who are interested in sex, of course, are admired and complimented as "studs").

Female children and teenagers are still taught that their self-worth depends to a large extent on being sexually attractive and desirable and on knowing how to "play the dating game." Meanwhile, boys are told that they should be "getting" (as in "getting a blow job" or "getting laid") rather than "giving" and sharing sexual pleasure.

And while women are supposed to have less interest in sex than men, they're still the ones who are supposed to be more responsible for contraception. But if they are, in fact, prepared, they are judged harshly and seen as "wanting it." No wonder it feels so crazy and confusing for adolescents, especially female adolescents; it's as if there is no way for them to win, to carve out a sane and sensible path toward healthy sexuality.

Over the years, I have had many families come to me asking for advice when their adolescent daughter has requested assistance getting birth control. One thing that often seems to be the case is that they're putting the cart before the horse and trying to address one question before other, more important, questions have been asked and addressed.

In your case, since you have known Dante for only several months, the most important question to put on the table for you and your family to consider is not "Can I get birth control pills?" but "What kind of relationship with Dante do I want, and how close to him do I currently want to be?"

As you probably know by now, sexual behavior involves not just sexual intercourse but any physical contact between two people who experience delight as a result of that contact. In this sense, hand-holding can be as sexual as oral sex, a peck on the cheek can be as sexual as French kissing, an arm around the shoulder can be as sexual as intercourse. What distinguishes these behaviors from each other is what they signify, what they mean, what they say about two individuals' relationship with each other.

In a way, you could imagine that all of these interactions occur across a broad spectrum, with the ones that require relatively little commitment, trust, maturity, and physical and emotional risk at one end (hand-holding, hugging, freak dancing); the ones that require relatively greater commitment, trust, maturity, and physical and emotional risk in the middle of the spectrum (French kissing, touching breasts and genitals through or without clothing); and the ones that require the greatest commitment, trust, maturity, and physical and emotional risk at the other end of the spectrum (intercourse, oral sex).

Often, when we're in a relationship, we're able to match up the nature of our sexual interaction with the amount of relational closeness that we desire, and things feel just right, with both partners comfortable and happy with how much of themselves they are sharing with each other.

Sometimes, however, for various reasons, individuals will make decisions about the nature of their sexual interaction that are out of sync with the amount of relational closeness they are seeking. At these times the relationship is put at risk and we become vulnerable to emotional pain.

What and how much we share physically in a relationship

is really not all that different from what and how much information we share in a relationship. While we might easily disclose our favorite book, movie, restaurant, or kind of music with just about anyone we found ourselves in a conversation with, we would only disclose more personal matters, such as our religious beliefs or home address or career plans, with someone with whom we had established some trust and closeness. And we would only share our deepest, most secret thoughts and feelings with someone in whom we had *complete* trust and confidence, who would never violate that trust and confidence by judging us or divulging these private thoughts and feelings to others without our permission.

What's also important to remember is that just as once you've disclosed an intimate secret to someone, you can't reverse the process and make believe it never happened or fully prevent him or her from betraying you, once you've engaged in a certain level of sexual behavior with someone, you can't reverse the process and pretend that it never happened—it changes forever the nature of your closeness with that person.

At times, of course, that is exactly what we want to happen, such as when we're in a relationship that is growing nicely, that is characterized by evolving kindness, trust, communication, and respect. Sometimes, however, the level of sexual behavior works against the relationship, with one or both partners regretting the steps toward sexual intimacy that were taken. At these times the relationship, as well as the two individuals in the relationship, suffer, and it becomes difficult to go back and reclaim the balance and comfort level that you had once enjoyed.

And that is what I want you to think about right now. If you are completely convinced that at this point in your relationship with Dante you are absolutely ready not only for the emotional and physical risks entailed by sexual intercourse (including pregnancy, because no birth control is foolproof) but also for the increased commitment to and closeness with Dante that will be the result, then you and your mother should meet with your gynecologist and look into the best form of contraception available (remembering—I'm sorry if I sound like I'm nagging you—that many effective contraceptives do not simultaneously prevent STDs). This doesn't mean that you *have* to engage in sexual intercourse, just that you've at least eliminated some of the risks of doing so should you eventually choose to.

However, if you have any doubts of any kind about taking this step, then without question it is better to be patient and wait and to tell Dante that you don't think you or the relationship is ready for the kind of sexual involvement that the two of you have been considering. Remember that the more time a couple gives a relationship to deepen and expand prior to becoming sexually active, the more enjoyable and meaningful sexual activity will ultimately be.

If you decide to wait and if Dante cares about you and the connection that the two of you have established, then he will respect your wishes and appreciate your honesty. If he doesn't, if he insists that despite your misgivings, the two of you should go ahead and have sex anyway, if he suggests that the future of your relationship with each other depends on this step being taken right now, then you'd really have to question the basis for your relationship with him and whether he might be more interested in using you than in loving you.

I know that this is a very complicated matter and that part of you might wish that I would just convince your parents to arrange for you to start taking the Pill and ignore all of this other stuff I've been focusing on, but as you know, I really want the best for you, and I care too much about you to keep my thoughts about this matter entirely to myself.

As always, even if we're in disagreement, let's see if we can keep things open and remain in contact.

Respectfully,
Dr. Sachs

16

Why Do I Do
What I Do?

—

Dear Amanda,

As you are aware, your parents gave me a call last Friday night when you were upset about not being allowed to go out with your friends because they didn't think you had cleaned your room to their specifications and because you were throwing things around the house and threatening to run away or harm yourself. Because these kinds of disturbing (for your mother and father) events have come up before, I found myself giving some thought to when they occur and came up with a hypothesis that I wanted to share with you.

I know that your father, as part of his work, travels a great deal and is often away from home for several days at a time at least once a month. I have heard from your mom that despite this routine having been in place for many years—since before you and your brother were born—she still finds it stressful when he's on the road.

As I looked over my notes, one of the things that I noticed was that none of these "Amanda-based" crises or emergencies ever occur when your dad is away from home. It's almost as if you're on your "best behavior" when it's just you, your brother, and your mother at home.

Just as interestingly, it was hard to ignore the fact that the crises and emergencies that *do* occur always seem to take place either just before your dad leaves on one of his trips or just after he has returned. Your dad even mentioned that himself when we spoke on the phone. He had just gotten back from four days of travel and commented to me, "Why do these things always have to happen right when I get home? I'm not in the house more than twenty-four hours before everything is exploding!"

Your mom once offhandedly mentioned this as well. I remember, during a meeting that you did not attend, her observation that she always dreaded the couple of days before one of your dad's trips because "that's when everything seems to go downhill—it's like an alarm goes off and it's Amanda's time to go ballistic."

Assuming there's some validity to this pattern, here is an explanation for what might be happening that I'd like you to contemplate. It is probably not a revelation to you that your mom and dad have had some ups and downs as a couple over the years. They have never separated and have never suggested to me that they think about doing so at this time, but there have been periods of time during which both of them have not been all that satisfied with each other and have wondered about the future of their relationship. They've told me that they've gone through phases where they don't share a bed together—something that they know you have noticed and commented on—and that is generally a sign that things are not going so well for a couple. You may remember mentioning this as well, in one of your first letters to me, when you wondered why your parents stay together when they so rarely seem to enjoy each other's company.

Now, your parents have been married for more than twenty years, and it's impossible to live together for that long without some ups and downs. I don't know what you imagine marriage to be like, but no husband and wife are pleased with each other all the time, and differences of opinion on matters ranging from money to work to child rearing to sex to in-laws always crop up, and go with the marital territory.

Some couples, when things get tense and difficult, find themselves fighting with each other more—it is as if their marriage becomes a battleground, with the smallest conflicts quickly escalating into all-out war. Other couples, when things get tense and difficult, do the opposite and pull away from each other—it is as if their marriage becomes a cemetery, with all of their complaints and grievances interred as they become more and more remote in an effort to avoid dealing with their conflicts.

From what I have seen, your parents fit more into the latter category than the former. And I believe that because you are so astute and such a dutiful daughter, you instantly sense the gap that starts to open up between them and reflexively, without even necessarily being aware of this, do whatever you can to bring them back together. In your case, I believe that what you have learned is that if you create a big enough crisis, your parents will suddenly find ways to overcome their distance and differences and move closer to each other so that they can figure out what to do with you. It's as if you once again find a way to sacrifice yourself, to give them a reason to come together during a period of time in which they may be feeling somewhat fed up with each other, and provide them with an opportunity to become a team, allies rather than enemies.

"What are we going to do with her?" and "What consequences do we need to impose?" become the questions they ask, ones that appear to rally them together, rather than, "Why does my spouse have to be so impossible?" or "Why did I marry him or her in the first place?"—questions that appear to keep them apart.

The funny thing is that your parents see your problems and crises as evidence of your *lack* of caring about them. "Why does she have to go crazy right before her dad leaves?" and "Why does she have to be so difficult the moment I return from a trip?" they ask, oblivious to your secret (secret even from yourself, I suspect) agenda. The reality as I see it, however, is that the process gets set into motion at this dependable frequency precisely because you *care so much,* because you feel compelled to do whatever you can to remind them of their partnership with and commitment to each other, to help them rediscover the reasons, the motivation, and the will to stay together, particularly when they're about to be apart for a while or have to figure out a way to adjust to being in each other's presence again.

So here's what I am going to propose to you. I think that you have carried the burden of trying to keep your parents together long enough, and although you have engaged in yet another act of self-sacrifice valiantly and without complaint, it's time to release yourself from the responsibility of doing so—it's heavy, it slows you down, and it's not really helping you or your parents anymore for you to continue to shoulder it. I would like to help you put down that burden, and to make it easier for you to do so, I am going to ask you to let me carry that burden *for* you for a while.

I have scheduled a few meetings with your parents without you so that they can begin to focus on and improve their relationship with each other as husband and wife, not just as father and mother, and to see if I can help them tune things up a bit. I can't give you a guarantee that I will be successful, and of course I don't have a crystal ball, but while I'm busy trying to give them a hand, I'd like you to back off for a while and give me a chance to do my job. In this case, backing off would mean freeing yourself from the commitment to come up with the crises and problems that are your calculated attempt to bring your parents back into the same orbit with each other.

I hope that you won't feel offended by my "firing" you from the job that you have taken on, and I'm not saying that you can never return to it or that you haven't done well at it—it's quite possible, in fact, that one of the reasons that they're still together is that you've provided them with some solid reasons to stay together. But while a good deal of your problematic behavior may originally have been designed to keep them committed to each other, it's simultaneously making it hard for them to move forward as a couple and really enhance their marriage. In other words, your efforts, devoted and well intended as they are, appear to have outlived their usefulness. Plus, what are they going to do when you have graduated and left home? They can't rely on you forever, you know.

So as (one more!) experiment, I'd like you, for now, to keep things as calm and settled as possible during the few days before your dad departs and the few days after his return, and let's see what happens.

Meanwhile, I'd also like you to give some thought to the general theme that we're discussing here, of which this issue is a specific example—I'm talking about your tendency to sacrifice and donate parts of your self to make things better for others, to display more fidelity and loyalty to others than to yourself. We've seen evidence of this in your relationship with Peter; in your relationship with your brother, Craig; and in your relationship with your parents. I wonder what would happen and how your life would feel different if you were a little more attentive to yourself and a little less attentive to everyone else.

Your curious clinician,
Dr. Sachs

17

Why Is Life So Painful?

—

Dear Amanda,

I was left speechless after reading your last letter, in which you told me that your friend Daryl had been killed in a car accident. It is always difficult to come to terms with *anyone's* death, but when it is the death of a young person, and the young person is a dear friend, the feelings of loss and pain can be almost too much to bear.

I certainly remember your mentioning Daryl in a couple of previous letters, how the two of you shared a "bizarre" sense of humor, how you worked together on the school literary magazine, how he had been there for you so many times when you were feeling lost and alone.

In your letter you were quite justifiably asking the question that all of us must ask when confronted with a reality that seems harsh, cruel, and unjust: "Why did this have to happen?"

The answer, unfortunately, is that no one knows. One of the most formidable challenges of growing up is being forced to encounter a world that does not always treat us, and the people who matter to us, very well. Sometimes the injuries that we are subjected to in life are temporary and we are able to recover from them fully with care and time. Sometimes, however, they last forever, leaving us with wounds that never completely heal. The skin of our world suffers a gash that is too gaping to be stitched up, and it remains as a constant reminder of the person who was so suddenly and heartlessly wrenched from our world.

Right now you are stunned and reeling, thrown into a grief that is deeper than one you have ever known before. This is as it should be, and nothing I say will or should pull you out of it. You are actually doing exactly what you are supposed to be doing, which is entering and experiencing the profound ache that accompanies great loss.

What I want you to remember, however, is that grief, painful as it is, does have a purpose to it—it unknowingly provides us with a path to follow through the interminable darkness that eventually brings us slowly, wincingly, back to the light. Of course, it takes great courage to grieve fully for what we have lost, and it is not a process that should be fixed, cured, stopped, or shortened.

But don't make the mistake of thinking that there is a particularly "right" or "wrong" way to deal with loss. Some people cry and some people don't; some people rage and some people don't; some people frequently mention the individual who has died, some people don't; some people go to the funeral or visit the grave site, some people don't. Everyone grieves in their own original way, and that way should be respected and accepted for what it is.

There is also no predictable timing or schedule to grief—the only real answer to the question "How long will I be mourning?" is "As long as you are mourning." That doesn't mean that you'll always be suffering as much as you are now, but it does mean that grieving is a lifelong process, one that changes over time but is never fully finished.

But however you grieve for Daryl, and however long it takes for you to do so, it is important to remember that grief that is utterly experienced is, ultimately, a process that deepens and awakens us, that liberates and illuminates us. We really don't know who we are until we have been hurt and have struggled bravely to make sense of that hurt and move on. A wise rabbi once wrote that "nothing is as whole as a broken heart." I think what he meant by this is that we're never really living our lives fully and completely unless we have experienced the despair that takes over when life breaks our heart.

Of course, you are probably, and understandably, thinking that you would gladly trade all of this wisdom and self-knowledge, all of this deepening and awakening and liberating and illuminating, if you could just have Daryl back in your life again, if you were able once more to cut his hair, to make him laugh, to torment his quirky dog, and to stay up late watching bad movies with him. But this, as you know, is not a trade that you have the power to make.

What you *can* do, however, is decide how you are going to keep your memory of him alive, how you are going to continue to embody what he stood for, and how you are going to allow this tragedy to transform you. This is not something for you to figure out how to do right now—right now is simply the time to accept and endure this unspeakable loss.

But ultimately the best way to go on living after we have encountered death, particularly a death that was so sudden and inexplicable, is to allow the loss to elevate us and uplift us. Viktor Frankl, a psychiatrist who survived the concentration camps during World War II, once wrote that "death gives life meaning." Your work is not to flee and become a fugitive from your grief but to allow the grief that you are feeling to wash over you and help you discover who you are and what about your life is most meaningful, most precious, most sacred.

Great pain cannot be avoided—it will always hunt us down and find us, no matter how cleverly we hide. But the lessons that great pain holds forth are always there for us; we may never welcome these lessons, but we can decide how they are going to change us and grow us up. All anguish has numerous treasures buried beneath it, and our job at these times is to dig up these treasures and bring them to the surface so that they have the possibility of enriching our lives and the lives of others.

There were some other issues and concerns that you expressed to me that I want to be sure to address in this letter. One is that you feel deprived because you never had a chance to say good-bye to Daryl, that he had been dead for hours before you heard what had happened. Surely one of the most upsetting aspects of this for you is that you were so ambushed by his death, that you didn't get the opportunity to share with him how much you cared for him, how much you valued him, how much you'll miss him, and all the other thoughts and words in your heart that you would have wanted him to hear.

With this in mind, here are a couple of things to think about.

First, I once read that what separates the living from the dead is not a wall but a window. While encountering the person that we have lost through a window is not the same as actually being able to *be* with him, it still allows us a glimpse and provides us with an undying connection that can comfort us and leave us feeling less alone.

Second, a patient of mine whose father had died once told me that she often used to dream about him at night but then wake up in the morning very sad, because as soon as she arose she was reminded that it had only been a dream and that he really wasn't there anymore as a part of her life. After a while, however, she learned to treat his visits to her dreamworld as a gift—an opportunity, however fleeting, to be together, to see him, experience him, love him, and miss him—rather than as a hurt.

I am telling you these things because even though Daryl has died, I don't believe it is too late for you to say good-bye to him. I think that you should assume that he is listening to you and that you should say all the things to him that you wanted to say and didn't have the chance to. Whether you do it in your head or in writing, by yourself or at the cemetery, you can still tell him how much he meant to you, how much he gave you, what you will never forget about him, what you want to thank him for, what you want to forgive him for or be forgiven for, and what he stood for and believed in that you will carry on for him for the rest of your own life. I think good-byes are very important, but I don't believe that a good-bye's importance is diminished in any way just because it is said after a person has already departed.

You also mentioned that you feel guilty, and that you were starting to think about cutting and carving yourself again in response to that guilt. Amanda, I don't know anyone who has lost someone important who doesn't feel some guilt, even if their relationship was basically a healthy and satisfying one, even if they had nothing at all to do with the loved one's death.

Sometimes it's easier or better for us to feel guilty than to acknowledge our powerlessness over the random way in which the universe seems to operate. That may be why you can't stop wondering what would have happened if you had invited Daryl over the evening of the accident—perhaps, if he had walked his dog over to your house and hung out with you instead of deciding to get in a car with his friend and go for a ride, the accident would never have occurred.

This kind of guilt—what is called irrational guilt, guilt that has no logical basis but that surely exists and has to be dealt with nonetheless—deceives us into believing that if we had just "done something" this terrible fate could have been averted.

There is also something known as "survivor's guilt," a kind of guilt that shows up when someone important to us has died inexplicably—we wonder why it was that *we* survived and *he* did not, why we were spared the tragic fate that our loved one succumbed to. Survivor's guilt is irrational guilt too—there are no substantive grounds for it; it just seems to be one of the methods we utilize to try to explain why something terribly inexplicable has happened.

So let me be clear with you about this, Amanda—I know that you feel some guilt about Daryl's death, but I want you to understand that you have no *reason* to feel guilty. You were not the cause of his death, and there would be no wisdom or purpose in your harming yourself or killing yourself in response to this dreadful fatality.

You may find that this guilt of yours eases over time. But should it not, you might want to try to find something to do that would help to take the edge off the guilt. Perhaps you want to visit the spot where the accident occurred and leave a flower or a note. Perhaps you want to invite your fellow friends and classmates to create a memorial for Daryl at the school. Perhaps you want to do something kind for his family, like visiting them during their period of mourning or baking them a loaf of bread or writing them a letter in which you remind them of all the things that made Daryl so special.

The point is that sometimes we are plagued by guilt that really isn't justified, and it's just not enough to try to talk or think ourselves out of these guilty feelings—instead, sometimes we have to *work* our way out of them and find a way to make the feelings useful. Once guilt has been channeled in a meaningful way and shown that it can have value and purpose, it usually stops afflicting us unnecessarily and can actually become a source of growth and change.

Finally, at the end of your letter you wrote that events like this "convince me that there is no God, because what kind of God would let a great seventeen-year-old like Daryl die, when so many other assholes go right on living?" In all the letters that we have written back and forth to each other in this past year, you and I have not yet addressed the matter of God, so I suppose now is as good a time as any for us to do so, and for that, I'm glad that you invited God into our conversation.

I wish that I could say that there is a divine force that is completely loving, just, and fair, that protected all who were good and punished all who were bad, but I've seen enough and learned enough to have given up on that belief a long time ago. I can tell you, though, that I believe in God anyway. And without getting into the specifics of my religious background, I can tell you that, from my perspective, while God did not keep Daryl from dying, God can be there for you as a source of comfort and strength as you mourn his mystifying death.

No one will be able to convince me that Daryl died because God needed to punish him or those who cared about him or because God "wanted" or "needed" him in heaven more than you or his family wanted or needed him on earth.

But I believe that God is there for you, and for all of his friends and family, to make everyone's suffering feel less lonely, to make everyone's pain feel less scary, to make everyone's faith feel less futile.

I cannot adequately explain to you why Daryl is dead—that is a tragedy that has no answer. But I can explain to you that the reality of death, however it comes, does not have to define and limit our life and how we live it. A car accident robbed you of the future that you could have had with Daryl, but it cannot steal from you all that you shared with him in the past or the ways in which you can keep his spirit, and your own, alive and flourishing forever.

As I said at the beginning of this letter, Amanda, it takes courage to grieve. You would not be feeling the intense pain that you are feeling right now had you not experienced the intense closeness with Daryl that both of you enjoyed. But your closeness has not died just because Daryl did—it can remain alive in important ways if you allow it to, if you continue traveling along the river of sorrow that you are currently in the midst of and cultivate on its banks the memory, dignity, and hope that will always be yours to cherish.

With deepest sympathy,
Dr. Sachs

18

Am I Really in Love?

Dear Amanda,

Of all the questions that we've been exploring over this past year, the one that you posed in your last letter—"Am I really in love?"—is one that everyone should be fortunate enough to ask at some point in their lives. Love, after all, expresses the yearning, the dream, the desire, and the wish that lie deepest in all of us. It is a force that animates, brightens, remakes, and rekindles our lives. It extends the horizons of our hearts in ways that no other encounter or experience ever can or ever will, and when love is recognized, felt, and shared with another person, it becomes the moment when we are not only most fully human but also most near to the divine.

Of course, because the longing to love and to be loved is so profound, the risks of love become profound as well. We are never as vulnerable as when we approach the threshold where two separate lives begin to engage and become intimate, when we entrust another person with our very souls and disclose our most private thoughts and feelings, and the journey of love is always an uncharted, unpredictable one that will eventually take us into some very perplexing and precarious waters. *Anything* can happen when we embark on this journey, and the possibility for hurt and misery is always distressingly close at hand. So with this much at stake, it's natural to think carefully about a new relationship and to try to get a sense of whether it truly embodies love.

As is the case with all of life's most pressing, urgent questions, "Am I in love?" can be answered only by you alone rather than by anybody else. To some extent, why, how, and with whom we fall in love will always remain an enigma, and nobody will ever be able to define love with much precision or establish with certainty whether you are "officially" in love. And when we are strongly attracted to someone, we usually find ourselves in a keenly emotional state that sometimes impairs our objective judgment and makes it difficult to see the other person, ourselves, and the relationship with much clarity.

To complicate things further, it's also quite easy to confuse love with other strong feelings that may be directly or indirectly related to love but ultimately are quite different and may even interfere with it. At various times, for example, we will all find ourselves confusing sexual attraction with love, jealousy with love, neediness with love, intensity with love, possessiveness with love, even, in some cases, mistreatment with love.

But despite the complexity involved with explaining love, perhaps I can help you to better address and answer your question by sharing some of my own thoughts and experiences on this matter.

The ability to love—to provide and accept care, warmth, support, tenderness, and affection—is life's highest achievement. But from my perspective, true love is best understood not as something that you have a certain quantity of or feel to a certain extent but by the *acts* of love that we display and observe. I always tell people that the best way to judge a loving relationship is by taking note of what they, as lovers, are doing rather than by what they are feeling or saying.

When two individuals behave in a way that makes it clear that their partner's needs and wants matter as much as their own, that is evidence of love. When two individuals are open, honest, and faithful *with* each other and, in the process, build trust *in* each other, that is evidence of love. When two individuals make each other smile, that is evidence of love. When two individuals can focus on their attributes and appeal and be tolerant of or even overlook their flaws and imperfections, that is evidence of love. When two individuals are kind to, supportive of, and generous with each other, that is evidence of love.

When two individuals disagree with each other but can see their disagreements as a strength rather than a weakness and find ways to good-naturedly compromise and resolve their disagreements, that is evidence of love. When two individuals remember that they are, indeed, *individuals* and can maintain a relationship in which both of their individualities are respected and preserved, that is evidence of love. When two individuals can count on each other and rely on each other in times both good and bad, that is evidence of love. When two individuals see their relationship as a joint adventure but still actively help each other to achieve their most precious personal goals, even if they are not the same goals, that is evidence of love. And when two individuals *listen* to each other—listen fully, patiently, attentively, in the way that all of us want to be listened to—that is evidence of love.

Another way to know if you are "really" in love is to look at what results from your experience of love. If you discover that you are living your life in a better, richer, more positive and productive way, there's a good chance that you're in love. If you find yourself more motivated to do all that needs to be done at school and at home, there's a good chance that you're in love. If you find yourself treating other people better and more responsibly—not just your boyfriend, but your parents, your friends, your teachers—there's a good chance that you're in love. If you find yourself feeling more energy, more optimism, more patience, more empathy, there's a good chance that you're in love. If you have the sense that your life has renewed or enhanced meaning, purpose, and direction, there's a good chance that you're in love.

And of course if you find yourself enjoying your time with Dante, looking forward to seeing him, sharing interests and passions, dreams and doubts, tears and laughter, hopes and fears—that, too, would strongly suggest that you are in love.

Being in love doesn't mean that you'll always be *feeling* in love, however. Even the best partnerships are not going to feel gratifying, stimulating, and wondrous every moment of the day, and there should be room in every healthy relationship for some amount of indifference, conflict, uncertainty, irritability, and boredom. But as long as these feelings do not predominate—as long as they are the exceptions rather than the rule—they, too, can be incorporated into the relationship rather than detract from it, and become interesting threads in the overall embroidery that the two of you are beginning to compose.

Often when somebody asks if they're "really in love," I believe the questions that are really being asked (or should be asked) are: "Is this relationship going to be *good* for me?" "Is this person that I'm attracted to *right* for me?" and "Are things going to last?" While I am unfortunately not clairvoyant and am unable to divine and depict your relational future with absolute certainty, I can share with you some realities that may help you to answer, with decent accuracy, these questions too.

The best predictor of the possibility of love is actually when two people *like* each other, when they have either already established a friendship or realize that they could easily *have been* friends with each other had they not become romantically involved. When that sense of warm, affectionate companionship is in place, love has the potential to take root and grow.

On the other hand, there are always warning signs in any developing, deepening relationship, and attending to these signs can be difficult when we're in the highly charged state of feeling ardently drawn to another person. But despite the challenge involved, you might want to be on the lookout for them nonetheless, because they will help you to prepare for your relationship's future and enable you, to some extent, to immunize yourself against unnecessary hurt and harm.

As I mentioned above, when it comes to relationships, it is generally how we act that matters a great deal more than how we feel. Trying to change another person and make him or her into someone that he or she is not is not an act of love. Frequent lies or lame, confusing excuses for where one was or what one was doing are not acts of love. Cutting off all other significant relationships and clinging to one's lover, or being asked to do so by one's lover, are not acts of love.

Being jealous of and threatened by a partner's other relationships with friends and family is not an act of love. Expecting your partner to always be there for you, to solve all of your problems and unfailingly make you feel better, is not an act of love. Feeling like you need to be drunk or high whenever you get together is not an act of love. Being required to do something that you are not completely comfortable with to "prove" your love is not an act of love. Repeatedly being hurt but being told that "it wasn't meant to hurt" or that "you're too sensitive, can't you take a joke?" is not an act of love. Verbal and physical abuse, under *any* circumstances, are not acts of love.

If you are already seeing or if you begin to see behaviors of this sort in yourself or in Dante, then you need to consider the possibility that maybe this relationship is not as based on love as you had initially thought and start to think of ways to address that or even consider ending the relationship.

Related to this, I want to make one final point. Although we all have our fantasies about the "perfect romance," I don't think there is only one destined partner, one special "soul mate" for each of us here on earth. I don't think that love "happens only once" and that if you blow it or if that love does not flourish and is unreturned and unrequited that you are doomed to lead a neglected, loveless life. Subscribing to this belief makes us more frightened, more tentative, and more insecure than we need to be and than is best for a healthy relationship.

I cannot guarantee that Dante will always be the primary love of your life, but I *can* guarantee that should your bond with him run its course at some point and come to an end, there will be other individuals with whom you can create a loving relationship if you maintain an open mind and an open heart. In fact, it is usually the sum of our many experiences with love—painful as some of them may be—that helps us to mature and gradually lays the groundwork for the love relationship that ultimately turns out to be the most satisfying and enduring of all.

As I said at the beginning of this letter, the question that you are asking is evidence that you are in the midst of encountering the most meaningful of human endeavors. For this alone, no matter how things turn out, you should be proud. I hope that you are gentle with yourself as your relationship with Dante unfolds and that you are able to follow its twists and turns with joy, courage, and self-respect.

Supportively,
Dr. Sachs

19

Will I Ever Feel Better?

Dear Amanda,

Thankfully, at least some of the questions you ask are easy to answer. So let me begin by crisply replying to the queries that you threw out in your last letter:

No, I have not given up on you.

No, I'm not sick of you.

No, things are not hopeless.

No, not all of my other patients are doing better than you are.

No, you are not disappointing me because you still feel suicidal at times.

No, I do not wish you would just go away.

I know that you had a very bad week, particularly bad because things had been looking up for the last several weeks and because you were beginning to feel that the hardest of times were now permanently behind you. I know that it's very frustrating for you that your feelings of dispiritedness and despair stubbornly return and still, at times, grip you by the throat and don't seem to let go. I know that you must feel exasperated by the fact that there remain periods of time when you don't believe things are ever going to feel right or good.

But just so you know, I'm not expecting you to be "the perfect patient," getting better and better every day without experiencing any setbacks and detours. We all like to envision healing as being akin to climbing a mountain, leaving our dark, flawed, and difficult places forever below us and eventually arriving at an elevated promontory that is permanently aglow with wholeness, peace, and contentment. Despite our wishes and fantasies to the contrary, however, the nature of healing, and of life in general, is irregular and uneven, always more like two steps up and one step back than forward step after irrepressible forward step. Hard as we may climb, there will always be some more climbing to do.

You needn't apologize for your struggles, because, as I've said before, your struggles are part of who you are, and it is how you embrace and manage them, not their presence or absence, that defines the person that you are becoming. With this in mind, I'm certainly not going to think any less of you if I hear that you've temporarily run aground, nor am I going to give up hope or abandon faith in your resilience and your ability to prevail just because you continue to hit a rough patch from time to time. None of us *find* our way without repeatedly discovering that we have *lost* our way and trying time and again to resolutely stumble back on course.

Your only duties at these times are to be kind to yourself, to accept the invitation to be quiet and still, to observe yourself and take careful note of what has been going on in your life that might be contributing to things becoming so difficult, and, should you choose to, to remain in touch with me so that we can map out the terrain of your growth together, with its mixture of peaks and valleys, deserts and oases, plains and forests.

Believing that these desolate times can be good for you, that they can build your character and make you into a better, deeper, more humane individual, is an almost impossible task when you're feeling as wretched as you probably are right now, so I'm not expecting you to celebrate yet another undesirable encounter with agony and alienation. But please do not forget that these very arduous times, when they are survived, are always times of great learning and insight too— they hold forth lessons that, painful as they may be, enable us to take ourselves more seriously and be more receptive, sensitive, and attuned to our own vulnerability and the vulnerability of others, lessons that teach us about the immortality of loss and love, that school us in the grace and grandeur of the human spirit.

I know that among other artistic ventures, you enjoy throwing pots on a potter's wheel. In some ways, you might try to imagine that these dismal phases that we all must face from time to time work on us similarly to how one works on clay—they lean on us and mold us, sometimes firmly, sometimes excruciatingly, but ultimately with the goal of making us softer, warmer, and more supple, better able to be shaped into something both useful and beautiful.

Thank you for continuing to take the risk of staying in contact, Amanda, even though you don't have what you would consider to be very good news to report. And, as I see it, despite how bad a week it was, there *is* good news in your willingness to acknowledge your hurt and offer me the opportunity to help convince you that your value does not reside so much in how you feel as in who you are.

Patiently,
Dr. Sachs

20

—

Why Can't I Be
More Like You?

—

Dear Amanda,

In your last letter, while thanking me for being of help and support to you during the time that we have worked together, you also wrote about wishing that you could be more like me and wondering why you're not. In this reply, I want to take a moment to address your "wishing" and your "wondering."

First of all, I'm happy to accept your gratitude and pleased to hear that you believe that our time together and our letter writing have been valuable. However, I can honestly take only a small amount of credit for your growth, since *you* have really been the one who is doing all the growing. I guess I see our relationship as similar to that between a coach and an athlete—the coach can try to instruct, inspire, and motivate, but ultimately he stands on the sidelines while the athlete goes out to compete on the playing field. So if you are feeling that you have changed and grown over this past year (and it's clear to me as well as to your family and to other people I've spoken to, such as your teachers, that indeed you have), then you've really got to keep bending and extending your arm far enough that you pat *yourself* on the back rather than me.

Also, you have to remember that this is a two-way street—while you may have learned a lot from me, I suspect that I've learned just as much from you. Your honesty, your courage, and your heroically unwavering capacity to persist in the face of obstacles and impediments without completely tossing in the towel have taught me a great deal. The very best thing about doing the work that I do is that every hour I am invited to accompany so many remarkable individuals on the journey down to their most luminous, inexpressible depths, and we *all* end up returning from our adventures in this invisible realm a little more sufficient and complete, a little more patient and tolerant of ourselves and others, and a little more aware and admiring of our preciously complex natures, our unique blends of light and darkness, gifts and burdens, strengths and weaknesses.

You are free to thank me for being there for you, but I am also free to thank you for being there for *me,* for so fearlessly inviting me to struggle with you toward wholeness and goodness, to discover the dreams, passions, mysteries, and desires that dwell, concealed, in the soul, and to voyage fearlessly—even recklessly at times—into the rushing tides of promise and possibility.

Regarding your wish to be more like me, I will take that as a compliment, coming from someone whom I like and respect so much, but I would prefer to put it in a different context. I think the reason you sometimes wish you could be more like me is that somehow when you are in my presence (even if that presence is a "literary" presence), you actually begin to become and enjoy *you*. Based on what I've learned about you over this past year, I strongly suspect that that feeling of becoming and enjoying yourself has been a somewhat rare occurrence, rarer than it deserves to be, and I hope that this is changing as a result of the mirror I hold up for you, a mirror in which you are somehow able to see yourself more positively reflected than you have before.

So when you are wishing that you could be more like *me*, what you may really mean is that the recognition and appreciation of your true, prized self somehow seem to show up a little more regularly and dependably when we are in contact with each other. And the important thing to keep in mind here is that you're perfectly capable of being and treasuring yourself even without having me around in direct or indirect form—it's just a matter of trying to absorb and incorporate the very positive feelings about you that I have tried to share with you until they become a fuller, better part of *your* nature. Sometimes, when adult patients have confessed that they think they're "in love" with me, what they're beginning to realize is that they're finally falling "in love" with themselves. Then it's just a matter of staying in love with themselves without needing to have me around to play Cupid and shoot my little arrows into their heart.

Regarding your wondering why you are not more like me, I'm sure you won't be surprised to hear me say that it's not your job to be like me; it's your job to be like *you*. It's very easy to idealize therapists and other trusted adults when you're in the throes of the catastrophes and calamities that you have been in the midst of confronting and to imagine that they have somehow been inoculated against similar adversity in their own lives.

The reality is that I, like just about every other healthy

adult that I have had the privilege of meeting or working with, have felt just as defeated, hopeless, demoralized, and inadequate as you sometimes do. Do not believe for a moment that it's possible to come near to oneself, to emerge as oneself, to be true to oneself, to *live* as oneself, without having been perched for much longer than one would have preferred on the dangerous ledge of gloom and despondency.

When I was a young man, I was in treatment with a therapist whom I admired greatly and who for a period of time was of significant help to me. But throughout our treatment together, he worked very hard to convince me that he "had it made," that he no longer suffered or struggled, that he had somehow found satisfying answers to all of life's most pressing questions and was now finally, blissfully "above it all" and completely free of despair and affliction. After a while my work with him became less and less helpful as I began to feel more and more inferior to him, as I continued to grapple and flounder while he calmly, and somewhat condescendingly, explained to me why I remained so troubled and miserable despite his best efforts to be of assistance.

Eventually (and, I believe, wisely), I decided to discontinue my work with him, despite my therapist's strong insistence that I ought to remain in treatment. Two interesting things then occurred. One, I instantly began to feel better, rather than worse, once I finished up—I think I was suffering less because I was suffering less *in comparison* with him, or at least in comparison with who I thought he was or who he wanted me to think he was. Which leads to the second thing: I learned a little later on, and completely coincidentally, that his personal life, which he had never hesitated to share the most glowingly positive things about, had fallen into disrepair and was, frankly, somewhat of a mess. He was not at all the completely confident, successful individual that he had wanted to appear to be and that I had chosen to believe in. I think, in retrospect, that he was so uncomfortable with himself that he had to use some of his patients as a reassuring yardstick to measure himself against and feel comforted by.

My reasons for sharing this experience with you are to help you to understand that no matter how much you may admire me, I'm essentially no different from you, so you really have no choice but to admire yourself too. There is much more that links us than separates us, and you are not to imagine for a moment that I've been secretly given a magic vaccine that prevents me from ever again encountering dejection and hardship.

Yes, I've had the advantage of having lived longer than you and have slowly, painfully built some of the self-confidence and self-respect that comes with realizing that life's blows may stun us but rarely annihilate us. You are free to emulate and strive toward developing those qualities, if you'd like, but you're *not* free to diminish yourself in the process of doing so—because you will surely see that you are able, over time, to build that same self-confidence and self-respect and to realize that you are a strong and capable survivor, as well.

In any case, whenever you find yourself looking up to me, I'd like you to think more about looking up to yourself. When you discover that you're wishing that you were more like me, I'd like you to wish that you were more like you. I may have helped to guide you onto the path toward change, but you are the one who's begun traveling it in your beautiful and unmistakable way. It is truly an honor to be in attendance as you gradually take up residence in your evolving adult self.

With gratitude,
Dr. Sachs

21

Whose Grief
Is This, Anyway?

—

Dear Amanda,

I was pleased that you have been continuing to give some thought to the theme of how self-sacrificial you tend to be, but particularly pleased with one of the questions that came to mind as you pondered this. You noted correctly that while we have discussed the ways in which you have sacrificed yourself for boyfriends, for your brother, for your father, and for your parents' relationship with each other, we haven't really examined if and how you sacrifice yourself for your mother. I have been pondering this as well and wanted to propose to you the following possibility.

Your mother, as you know, basically had to finish growing herself up without a mother of her own. I learned from her that your maternal grandmother died when your mother was only thirteen and her two younger brothers were ten and eight. As sometimes happens in situations like this, one child takes on a parental role, and your mom essentially became a mom herself at the age of thirteen, entrusted with the responsibility of keeping an eye on your two uncles while her dad, your grandfather, continued working full time and trying to make ends meet.

Your mother sacrificed a great deal, herself, during those years. She told me, and may have told you as well, that she was unable to participate in many junior high and high school activities or have much of a social life because of the family commitments that she was asked, and felt compelled, to uphold.

And while your grandfather eventually remarried, his new wife wasn't all that interested in being a stepmother— she had also been widowed, had two children of her own, and didn't provide much support or warmth to your mother and her brothers. It was probably a little easier on your mom once her father married again, but the new family that was created as a result was apparently not a very caring or comforting one, and isn't even to this day.

Your mom seems to me to have labored to come to terms with the loss of her mother since the day she died. Losing a parent when you are still a child, as I'm sure you can imagine, causes pain and sorrow that reverberates for decades—indeed, your whole life.

Now, one thing you surely know that I have tried to communicate to you throughout our correspondence is the fact that human behavior never takes place in a vacuum. How we think, how we feel, and how we act are the result not only of what is occurring inside of us but also of the interactions that are occurring between us and those that we are close to. Who we are and what we do are always at least partially a response to who others are and what others do. It's like a very sensitive feedback loop, in a way, with each one of us making moves that trigger responses in others, responses that in turn trigger counterresponses in us, on and on and on.

This feedback loop is particularly complicated when it is taking place between members of different generations within a family. For example, it is very common for us to think about and acknowledge the ways in which our genetic heritage influences, to a large extent, many of our physical characteristics. You already know that specific individual traits such as hair color, height, cholesterol level, and predisposition to cancer have been shown to be the result of what has been passed on to us by our forebears.

But it is just as true that our *psychological* heritage influences, to a large extent, our emotional characteristics and our subsequent behavior. This linkage may not be as easily revealed or identified as a physical one, but it exists nonetheless. In a way, this psychological heritage is kind of like gravity—which is invisible, but we know that it is real based on what results from it, such as apples dropping to the ground rather than sailing toward the sky, or planets revolving in fixed orbits around stars rather than flying randomly off into space.

So what does this have to do with you and your mother? In your case, I believe that the psychological heritage that your mother passed on to you is carried by the tremendous waves of sadness and emptiness that rose up within her after her mother's death and that have been repeatedly pounding, since you were born, onto your own shores. I don't think that your mother planned on passing these waves on to you—I doubt that she even knows that she's been doing it.

But parents always, to some extent, turn to their children, the next generation, to compensate them for old losses, to heal their old wounds, to make them feel better, more complete, and more whole. Somehow, I believe that your mom instinctively knew that becoming a mother would help her to better bear the loss of her own mother. But because her feelings of loss were buried under the responsibilities that were thrust upon her as a young woman, she, just like your father when his sister, your Aunt Delia, died, was never given the opportunity to grieve this loss.

And this, conveniently, is where you come in. I think that you, through a combination of volunteering for and being assigned to this role, became the "designated mourner" for your mom, the one who tacitly agreed to take on the role of crying the tears that she was never able to cry.

When we were exploring the connection between your father's relationship with Aunt Delia and his relationship with you, I told you how all parents are instantly on the lookout for ways to identify with their children so that their children become more familiar to them and thus easier to make a commitment to. Similarly, adolescents, as part of their growing up, will often look for ways to identify with their parents, to make sense of their mother and father, particularly their same-sex parent.

So when you wonder what you may have been sacrificing for your mom, it could be that you have been willing to take on your mother's grief, agreeing to become its envelope and container as a gift to your mom, who needed some help and some company after having managed it mostly by herself for so many years.

And while you've been very generous to offer her this gift, the problem is that it doesn't really work to anybody's advantage anymore—it keeps your mom from ever addressing and healing her grief because she's so distracted by having to deal with your difficulties, and it burdens you with a grief that was never really yours to carry.

Some of the great sadness that you have been wrestling with these last few years is surely yours, and yours alone, but some of it is just as surely your mom's, growing out of your deep sense of duty to her and an equally deep desire to protect, connect with, and understand her. In a sense, you have become both like your mother, mourning her losses for her, and like your grandmother, trying to comfort your mother like a loving parent does, by helping her to carry the weight of her sorrow. No wonder you sometimes feel so overwhelmed.

Now, a little mothering of one's own mother is appropriate and healthy. But it appears to me that you've been doing a *lot* of it, far too much for your own good, and just as important, far too much for your mother's good. One thing that every young adult has to learn is the difference between giving care and taking care of. Unless someone is fully dependent on us, such as a baby or an individual with a serious handicap, it is better to learn to give care than to take care of, because "taking care of" someone always diminishes us and the person that we're trying to take care of and prevents both of us from growing.

I think that you have been tuned in to your mother's emotional issues your whole life, whether you or she has known it or not. But *you* are not *her,* and you are not her mother—she is *your* mother. I wonder if the roles have gotten a little mixed up over the years and if reestablishing and clarifying them might not be a good thing for everyone involved.

Amanda, I have noticed that you have been chiming in a good deal more frequently in our last few family sessions, and I'm hoping this is a sign that you are feeling more comfortable speaking up and contributing and are seeing some value in doing so. With this in mind, I thought it might be a good idea for me to schedule a meeting with just you and your mom to talk some of these matters over. Sometimes, when unhelpful patterns have been in place for a long time, you have to chisel away at them bit by bit to break them so that new and better patterns can grow to take their place.

I will look forward to seeing what new sculpture we can chisel out for you and your mom so that you are both liberated from a prison that neither of you need remain in any longer.

Optimistically,
Dr. Sachs

22

Why Am I Here and Where Am I Going?

DEAR AMANDA,

I can tell that this will be one of the last in-depth letters that I will be writing to you, for several reasons. One, you've begun more actively participating in our individual and family sessions, engaging much more naturally with your parents and with me, so there's less need for us to write to each other between sessions. Two, things seem to be pretty steadily improving for you now, not without some steps sideways and backward, but certainly with some significant overall forward movement.

Finally, the two-part question that you brought up in your most recent letter—"Why am I here and where am I going?"—suggests to me that you're doing what you need to

do to unhook from the past and that you are accurately sens-
ing that it's time to look ahead to your future. That's the
surest way I know that therapy is beginning to come to an
end and that a patient is ready to test her wings and begin
soaring away on her own.

This is not to say that these two questions are any easier
to answer than some of the others that you've been posing
over this last year. In fact, I have found that ultimately we become who we are meant to be more by asking questions
than by actually being able to answer them. But it's hard to
live without at least taking a stab at these big queries, so here
are some thoughts that you might want to keep in mind as
you begin to go in search of your answers.

While many would have you believe otherwise, I have
not found it to be the case that we ever maintain the ability
to clearly envision the path our lives will follow. In fact, I'm
never absolutely certain that there *is* a path—our life's journey seems more akin to setting sail across a vast ocean, with
an infinite number of directions and possibilities, with only
our passions and creativity, our imagination and intuition
there to guide us.

At times we will find ourselves sailing along smoothly
and effortlessly, as if we were following a clear, reliable map,
making steady progress toward our desired destination. At
other times the map will seem to have mysteriously melted
away, and we will feel adrift and astray, staring longingly
at the stars and horizon for even a vestige of navigational
guidance.

Ultimately, though, while you should not count on
being given a guide that will neatly chart your life's destiny,
you *can* trust that if you try very hard to attend carefully to
who you are, your voyage will always be illuminated, and it
will carry you both to many of the places that you have always dreamed of and to some unforeseen places that you

have never dreamed of but that await you with important and exciting possibilities nonetheless.

That is the essential drama of our plunge into life's wide and unpredictable waters, to find a way to fully become our selves, to be faithful to ourselves, to inhabit ourselves, and to discover how to uphold our own distinct nature while still participating in, sharing with, and belonging to the world.

As you surely have begun to figure out, however, from observing your own life as well as the lives of those around you, this drama does not always play itself out in jubilant and rewarding ways. Many individuals, despite their best, most devoted efforts, wind up living as if estranged from their own being, exiled from their own presence, breaking promise after promise to themselves, held hostage by the expectations of others, their most cherished desires concealed under dilapidated layers of obligation, obedience, and drudgery. The roads that would carry us to fulfillment and delight can be tricky and treacherous ones, with numerous potholes and obstacles littering the way, threatening to throw us completely off course.

Maintaining our integrity and remaining true to ourselves under the intense pressures to compete and conform that we are all susceptible to can be grueling indeed. It is no wonder that many wind up living their lives in hiding, escapees from the province of their own potential, eventually cut off almost completely from who they are and who they might become, from any knowledge of how to ignite the embers of their most heartfelt ambitions, dreams, longings, and wishes and fan them into a heat-giving fire.

So how do you take up residence in your innermost self and continue to travel toward your unique True North? The solution (and, it goes without saying, easier said than done) lies in allowing yourself to be still, silent, and attentive enough that your quietest music slowly becomes audible, that your innermost voice can begin to be heard, that you can engage in an intimate conversation with the most essential and eternal parts of yourself, because it is only as a result of that conversation that your life will be lived meaningfully and purposefully.

The reason this is easier said than done is that our modern culture invites, supports, and honors this important dialogue less and less as we become more and more enamored with other, less substantive and enduring matters that have very little to do with living soulfully. The force field that we all reside in—the one that insists that we *are* what we *have,* that more and faster is better than less and slower, that external gratification is more consequential than internal richness, decency, and dignity—presents a tremendous challenge to the discovery of our true colors, our true passions, and our true powers.

But no matter where and when you exist, the song of your soul is always being sung, even if, at times, in the faintest of whispers, and your task is to shut out as much of the outer world's noise as you can so that you are able to pay close attention to that which plays, radiant, inside you. When you do so, you will find, over time, that that is how your greatest discoveries, accomplishments, surprises, and triumphs will shine through.

The poet Rainer Maria Rilke once wrote of having "faith in the night," and I think that what he meant by this is that he had an abiding trust in what was darkest, that our blackest "nights" need not be fearfully avoided or frantically lit up but instead can be allowed to gently overtake us so that we can learn to see in the dark and to decipher the beauty and promise that calmly, faithfully reside there.

Of course, it's a much greater risk to travel the territory of the dark rather than the light, precisely because its geography is so much less visible, safe, and predictable—that is why so few people regularly do so. But it is *only* by doing so that your most interesting and authentic trails will be revealed to you and you will most surely be able to successfully engage with the questions that you so boldly put forth.

You have complained numerous times about feeling that you're "strange," "weird," and a "wing nut," and that can be a very difficult thing. Whenever we are distinct and separate, in whatever ways, we feel lonely and vulnerable, cut off from others and stranded. To my way of thinking, however, feeling "strange" is an experience that is absolutely crucial to awakening to yourself and forging a singular, original life. Recognizing and maintaining some "strangeness," some eccentricity or individuality, is your guarantee that you have not completely succumbed to all the larger influences that interfere with the ongoing task of getting to know yourself. Instead of feeling ashamed of and embarrassed by how different you feel you are from everybody else, you might try to celebrate that differentness, to see it as a compass that can guide you away from the perils of slavish conformity, from having your hardest, brightest edges filed drearily away.

Your creative spirit, Amanda, which expresses itself in so many ways, such as through your artwork and your writing, will be your most powerful ally in sustaining you on this journey through unknown (and sometimes unknowable) landscapes. The surest way to integrate our sense of being strange and welcome our odd or neglected parts is by allowing ourselves to be led by our imagination, because our imagination values, cherishes, and depends on being strange. For better or for worse, and at various points in your life it will feel more like one than the other, creativity will insistently call you forth, sometimes to a life that is abundant with adventure, vitality, and grandeur, sometimes to a life that is characterized by danger, vulnerability, and rejection. You cannot live a creative life without risk, constantly free from feelings of pointlessness, rejection, failure, and instability.

One way or another, though, your creativity is one of your greatest gifts—you will be able to (and sometimes will *want* to!) run from it, but you will never be completely able to hide from it. It will always beckon you back to your personal underworld, to the inner realms that glimmer with fantasy, dream, and wonder, and it will always remind you that nothing of significance is ever completely closed off to you.

And while you cannot live a creative life without risking failure, the risks of living without creativity are far more substantial and damaging. You consign yourself to being an inmate in the penitentiary of your own unexplored life, forever saddling your future with the inestimable weight of regret and trying to forgive yourself for this heartless crime against your own humanity.

One further thought to contemplate—you know that a significant theme that we have been exploring throughout the time that we have worked together is your very strong tendency toward self-sacrifice. I believe strongly that our most important accomplishments are the ones that not only feel right for us but also make a difference in the world, the ones that are both life-*living* and life-*giving*. Knowing you, it wouldn't surprise me if you were concerned that the ways in which I'm inviting you to answer the questions having to do with why you are here and where you're going—to dive as deeply as you can into your own invisible and sacred depths—will lead you to a life of isolation and selfishness. But you will find that a pilgrimage of this sort will yield a harvest that can feed not only your own soul but the soul of our entire planet. It may seem paradoxical, but it is when we are most intimately connected with ourselves—when we are *being* as much as we are *doing*—that we find ourselves most intimately connected with others.

One can never view others with more sensitivity and compassion than one is willing to view oneself with. With this in mind, Thomas à Kempis wrote, "First keep the peace within yourself, then you can also bring peace to others." Civilization's most selfless individuals did not become that way by abandoning and sacrificing themselves but by dauntlessly exploring every corner of their being and bringing the abundance that they found back from their depths so that they could better enrich the lives of the rest of us. In the final analysis, you will find, it's not what you have and what you do but who you are and how you love that will make for a real and meaningful life.

Amanda, you have grown and changed in unmistakably wondrous ways in the time that I have known you, and it has truly been an honor for me to bear witness to your remarkable transformation. I want you to know and believe that you are going to continue to grow and change in the coming years, sometimes in expected and sometimes in unexpected ways, and that with each stage you will surely develop a deeper, firmer sense of who you are and who you are destined to become.

But you will never be a finished product—we are forever works in progress (although sometimes more "work" than "progress") and we always have some evolving to do—that is what keeps us vital and human, perpetually brisk and alive with opportunity.

I know, through our spoken and written dialogues, that you have already begun acquiring the wisdom that the world is more question than answer. I hope you will always ask the kinds of questions that you have been asking over and over again throughout your years, and I hope that you will always be wrestling with and troubled by these questions, too, because that is how you will know that you are still growing. Nothing that is truly worth knowing can ever be taught—the most important questions will, at the end of the day, have to be *lived* rather than answered, but in living these questions we open ourselves up to that which is most essential, most valuable, and most infinite.

I will look forward to seeing where your journey takes you and to having the chance, from time to time, to continue to get a glimpse of the new and exciting life chapters that your indomitable spirit will surely author.

With affection and the greatest respect,
Dr. Sachs

EPILOGUE

When you share your sorrows,
you cut them in half.

−KOREAN PROVERB

My primary job as a clinician, as I see it, is to make myself obsolete and irrelevant, to provide the necessary guidance, perspective, and support such that my patients are liberated to resume sound, vigorous progress on their own, without needing me as the catalyst, the enzyme that sparks revival and rejuvenation.

I don't believe that psychological treatment should be an interminable process, and I do believe that there are *many* ways for people—children and adults—to understand their suffering, resolve their conflicts, heal their pain, and continue to embark on the hard but necessary work of growth that don't involve being in therapy.

As these last few letters suggest, Amanda slowly grew to trust the therapeutic process and began to more willingly participate in our sessions, so our letter writing became less

necessary and our correspondence gradually dropped off—
she had other, more important, people to build bridges with
besides me. And as Amanda and her family gradually pulled
themselves out of the quicksand they had been marooned in,
we scheduled our consultations less frequently.

This is not to say that this resilient young woman went
on to complete a euphoric, problem-free, and confusionless
adolescence. We eventually established a routine of rotating
sessions as she moved into her senior year of high school, in
which I met with Amanda and her parents once a month and
with Amanda alone once a month. During these sessions
there was usually something important that needed to be
teased out and dealt with.

Amanda did maintain her dependence on pot and alcohol to a greater extent than I would have preferred, a topic
that we addressed with regularity. She eventually chose to
break up with Dante on her terms, but only after (and probably because) they had become sexually active. This was followed by a period of allowing herself to become sexually
manipulated by and involved with several different young
men during her last months of high school.

That was one of the reasons I maintained an effort,
throughout our work together, to restore and rebuild some
of the closeness that she and her father had once enjoyed,
because I was speculating that she was looking to her male
peers to compensate for what had diminished between her
and her dad. However, it should be noted that Amanda did
accrue enough self-respect to always take the steps necessary to prevent any unwanted pregnancies and STDs despite her sexual activity, and that the boys she became
serially involved with were, for the most part, fairly solid
and reputable young men.

But overall, the progress that we did make in reformatting the grim equilibrium that she and her family were entrenched in when they first came to meet with me paid off handsomely. Once the ungrieved-for ghosts from the parents' painful past—specifically the deaths of Amanda's father's sister and Amanda's mother's mother, and the miscarriages that preceded her older brother's birth—were brought out into the open and exorcised, they were then able to be more fully mourned and integrated and subsequently lost the power to vandalize and jeopardize Amanda's and her family's future.

Amanda's parents met with me as a couple for about a dozen sessions, made some tangible improvements in their marriage, and chose to commemorate their twenty-fifth anniversary by renewing their vows, a ceremony that Amanda contributed a beautiful poem to. The poem was, to my way of thinking, a literary declaration of independence in which she was able to affirm her emancipation from the mission of saving her parents' marriage, because they had clearly taken over the task of saving it themselves.

Craig left home for college but experienced a very bumpy first year, partying too much, missing too many classes, winding up on academic probation, and finally returning home after his first semester of sophomore year. This was difficult for the family but certainly helped to loosen Amanda's previous stranglehold on the self-sacrificial, family-scapegoat role. It also meant that Craig had an opportunity to reduce the extent to which he had been sacrificing *himself*, in his case a sacrifice that had been regularly taking place on the altar of purity and perfection. With this in mind, I scheduled a few productive family sessions with all four of them to try to solidify the family's newly evolving and more flexible homeostasis.

And as Amanda herself was finally freed to unplug herself

from so much self-sacrifice, she found that she had enough energy at her disposal to pursue more growth-promoting activities and ambitions. She was named editor of the school literary magazine, she started taking photography classes at a local arts center, she reinvested in her academic work and began thinking about applying to college, she obtained her driver's license, and she got a job as a hostess at a local restaurant, providing her and her parents with further evidence of her burgeoning independence. She also began bringing samples of her art and creative writing into our sessions for us to discuss and explore together.

Not surprisingly, as she began to find that there might be valid reasons to focus on living rather than dying, there were no further suicide attempts, hospitalizations, or acts of self-mutilation.

In the spring of her senior year, Amanda gained acceptance to one of the universities that she was hoping to be admitted to, at which point we "formally" ended our therapeutic relationship with a couple of farewell sessions. I did stay in touch with her through e-mail and letters once she started college and, when some conflicts arose, encouraged her to consult with a clinician at the university's counseling center, which she agreed to do and which turned out to be helpful. In the meantime, I also set up several appointments with her brother and parents to address some age-appropriate difficulties that Craig was experiencing.

Amanda graduated from college with a major in studio art, got a job as a photographer and graphic artist for an advertising agency, and found an apartment with her boyfriend of two years. Her relationship with her parents improved significantly once she left home, and she remained attentive to and involved with them, and with her brother, without resurrecting too many of her messianic proclivities. She also volunteered to become a Big Sister, and finally swore off pot and alcohol.

Interestingly, after little more than a year at the ad agency, Amanda got back in touch with me to tell me that she had decided to apply to graduate school to earn a master's degree in clinical social work. This made me hark back to a sage comment a supervisor of mine had once made, that a healthy person is someone who can turn her preoccupation into her occupation. Amanda, who to my way of thinking had for so long been preoccupied with taking care of others through self-sacrifice, had masterfully figured out a way to make a *living* taking care of others, without losing her own life in the process.

With her having made the arduous journey from patient to healer, I am certain that her *own* patients will now be the fortunate beneficiaries of her courage, empathy, and wisdom.

———

Engrave this upon your heart:
there isn't anyone you couldn't love
once you heard their story.

—MARY LOU LOWNACKI

A NOTE TO TEENS

As you surely know by now, adolescence is a time of profound and irreversible change. It is as if you were being ripped away from the "who" that you were to become a sudden stranger not only to those who are familiar with you but to yourself as well. While there are some things about you that will stay essentially the same during this transformation, many of the ways in which you had previously come to identify yourself during childhood begin to evaporate, to be replaced by new and different thoughts and feelings, concerns and dilemmas, attributes and qualities, many of which you will not understand at first. While all of these will eventually become a part of you and turn out to be quite valuable, this process will nonetheless leave you, for an uncomfortably long period of time, feeling alienated and uncomfortable—disordered and disorganized, unbalanced and unrecognizable.

As I explained to Amanda, adolescence is a painful time largely because it represents a death: the death of childhood, with all its hopes and illusions. When someone important to us has died, our task is both to hold on and to move on—we must hold on to what we loved about that person so that we will always be comforted and inspired by our memory of him or her but simultaneously let go enough that we can move on with the rest of our lives without being burdened by who and what we have lost. The process of maneuvering through adolescence is ultimately the same—we need to hold on to those parts of ourselves and our families that deserve to be honored, cherished, and preserved but let go of the parts that we have outgrown so that we can move on with the delicate process of becoming a new, separate, and unique person.

This process is an unavoidably turbulent one, but this turbulence does have an underlying and timely purpose—it churns up the initiative, courage, energy, and resourcefulness to successfully mark and make the important passage into young adulthood. Because of this, I tend to worry more about the teens who are *not* experiencing this turbulence than those who are, because that suggests that they're not engaged in the psychological toil necessary to prepare for and embark on this journey. Most of the time the distress that my adolescent patients tell me about, real as it may be, is actually not the result of what's *wrong* with them but, rather, what's *right* with them.

In a way, it's sort of like chicken pox—when small children acquire chicken pox, it is an annoying but ultimately harmless illness that has the benefit of inoculating them against getting chicken pox for the rest of their lives. But if you don't fall prey to chicken pox as a child, you may always run the risk of succumbing to it as an adult, and chicken pox for an adult is *not* innocuous—at that stage of life it becomes a serious, potentially fatal disease. In other words, there are clear advantages to experiencing certain conditions at certain "seasons" in our lives, when we are best equipped to handle them.

As I mentioned in the prologue, you may not have had to deal with all or even some of the specific challenges and difficulties that Amanda was encountering, and your behavior may not be, become, or have been as worrisome and problematic as hers. But it is still impossible to ferry yourself from the shores of dependent childhood to the shores of self-reliant adulthood without encountering certain hazards along the way, and I am hopeful that much of what I offered to Amanda has some relevance and meaning for you as well, as you set sail across these vast and perilous waters.

Of course, there are many other ways to find strength, hope, and guidance besides reading this book. Making sure that you have dependable people to talk to is of immeasurable importance, and it's usually best if your personal support group comprises a combination of friends and trusted adults. And it doesn't have to be a throng, either—having one or two close friends and one or two solid adults is usually enough.

There are also professionals whom you can always turn to for assistance. Whether it's a special teacher or a coach, your guidance counselor or your family doctor, a member of the clergy or a therapist, you shouldn't ever hesitate to touch base with someone who is skilled at helping teenagers make sense of the disorientation they inevitably face.

You are probably already aware of the many growth-promoting, stress-reducing activities that are fruitful to engage in: exercise, prayer, meditation, creative expression, communing with nature, adopting good eating and sleeping habits, and other endeavors of this sort all help us to stay afloat in powerful currents.

You have seen in these pages that much of my work with Amanda, and many of my letters to her, focused on her role within, and the influence of, her family. It is important for you to remember during this stage of life that adolescence does not happen just to you, the adolescent, but also to your entire social world, of which your family is the most important component. That is why I spent much of my clinical "face time" with Amanda and her family together, as I do with most of the adolescents I work with.

With this in mind, it's always useful for you to take a look at your own relationship with your family, to see if you can determine the many ways in which you affect them and they affect you. Rather than simply blaming yourself or your parents or your siblings for behaving in the way that you all do, try to look for the "feedback loops" that perpetually exist. If you believe that your parents are too protective of you, for example, give some thought to what you might be doing that seems to elicit their protectiveness, or simply ask them what you might do to help them feel more trusting and less invasive. Invite them to share with you the basis for their level of protectiveness and what things were like for them when they were growing up that might account for their current style of parenting.

Sometimes it takes an outside observer, such as a family therapist, to make sense of certain interpersonal patterns and help to change them when they're not particularly healthy, but many times we are able to do this ourselves, simply by watching and listening carefully.

Finally, try to gently keep in mind that no matter how

hard you work, no matter how good you try to be, no matter how smart you are and how much awareness and insight you cultivate, you simply cannot live a life of fullness and vitality without experiencing pain. Suffering will always find its place in our lives, and the more respect and tolerance we display toward it and the more we attempt to learn from it, the less greedy and selfish it becomes and the less space it will need to inhabit.

I remember, back when I was a teenager and had first gotten my driver's license, that my mother would lend me her big brown Oldsmobile so that I could drive into the city where I had a part-time job. I'd have to take the expressway to get downtown, and it seemed that I always wound up in the one lane of the expressway that had numerous potholes and remained stuck in that lane because traffic was usually too snarled for an inexperienced driver like me to easily make a change.

So, swearing and sweating, I'd hit crater after crater, mile after mile, and each time the Oldsmobile would violently clunk and shudder and I'd be certain that I was destroying my mother's car, that it would suddenly collapse into a heap on the highway, leaving me stranded and my parents angry with me.

"Why can't I ever remember to get in the lanes that don't have the potholes?" I'd angrily ask myself, journey after frustrating journey. "Am I *always* going to make the same mistake over and over again?" It wasn't until I'd been driving back and forth for several months that I realized that *every* lane of this highway was filled with potholes. My point, as I'm sure you've figured out, is that every lane of life has its potholes, and there's no way to escape or avoid them if you ever want to get somewhere.

I once read that it is better to suffer and be wise than to

be tranquil and a fool. I hope that my letters to Amanda help you to make sense of your suffering, to increase your wisdom, to tolerate your flaws and imperfections, and to safely navigate the impressive and passionate passage that you are now in the midst of making.

——

Only the incomprehensible gives any light.

—SAUL BELLOW

A NOTE TO PARENTS

Nothing tests a parent's emotional mettle like raising a teenager. Adolescence always entails a profound upheaval, with teens laying a long, bruising siege to the family's carefully constructed foundation as they struggle to find a way to become their own person without losing their sense of belonging. Meanwhile, it is as if they release themselves into an orbit around the dark side of the moon, impossible to influence or communicate with effectively, while simultaneously refusing to offer any concrete, convincing evidence that they are ever going to return. And the times that they are actually needing us the most are the times when they are the least pleasant to be with, because they experience so much shame and chagrin about their neediness and manage their disappointment in themselves by becoming bristly and belligerent.

In my previous book, *The Good Enough Teen: Raising*

Adolescents with Love and Acceptance (Despite How Impossible They Can Be), I describe in detail the many ways in which this stage of life essentially constitutes a psychological tsunami that dramatically lifts the entire family out of the comfort of what has hitherto been reliable and ingrained and deposits them into a new, alien, and unanticipated habitat.

While a comprehensive summary of this complicated conversion is beyond the scope of this section, parent readers of this book may benefit from having a few important points highlighted.

A Yiddish proverb wryly notes that "small children bring headaches, but big children bring heartaches." Nothing can make parents feel more helpless than watching their teenager begin to run aground, particularly when the consequences of mistakes and errors at this stage of life are potentially so grave and irreversible.

But it is important to remember that the lens we choose to look at our children through determines to a large extent what we see, how we treat them, and who they eventually become. By the time Amanda's parents had come to meet with me, they were completely demoralized; despite having consulted with many well-intentioned clinicians over the years, they had eventually become certain that their daughter was psychologically defective, the hapless victim of innate emotional and neurochemical flaws that, at best, could be coped with but never fully resolved. As a result, they had understandably begun to segregate and isolate themselves from having any real impact on or responsibility for their daughter's welfare.

As I explained to Amanda in several of my letters, however, our behavior never occurs in a vacuum but is always influenced and engendered by those around us. It was my belief that Amanda's troubles were rooted not within her but within the system she was growing up in.

This is not to say that Amanda's parents were to blame for her difficulties—blame, to my way of thinking, has no place in family treatment. But it was important for everyone in the family to understand that while no one was to *blame,* everyone was *responsible* for their contributions to the family process of which Amanda's disturbing, self-destructive acts were merely a symptom.

When I was in graduate school, a professor of mine proposed that any adolescent suicide attempt has a genesis rooted in at least three generations, and his hypothesis seems well supported by Amanda and her family. The many layers of sorrow and loss that were substantially deposited well before Amanda was even born became the foundation for her own feelings of sorrow and loss—she intuitively picked up on her parents' suffering and rose to the occasion, trying futilely, without even knowing how or why, to ease it.

In *The Good Enough Teen* I proposed that the behavioral problems that adolescents display perform the function equivalent to that of canaries in a mine shaft—signifying when (emotionally) toxic fumes are leaking and need to be dealt with and neutralized before any further damage ensues. As I worked with Amanda and her parents, it became more and more evident that she was trying awkwardly, even dangerously, to alert her parents that there was some old and painful business that needed to be attended to if they were going to avoid further emotional danger and be authorized to once again move forward. While it was tempting to see her efforts as ineradicable signs of psychopathology, and her previous clinicians had apparently surrendered to that temptation, I believe that that approach would have been completely misguided.

The problem was not with Amanda but with the self-sacrificial missions that Amanda had been recruited to take on—carrying her parents' ancient grief for them, playing the scapegoat role to protect her brother and promote his regal standing, and attempting to save her parents' marriage—all of which were, quite simply, overwhelming and impossible to fulfill. It seemed to me that she was not so much *de*pressed as *op*pressed, suffocated by the family duties that she was submitting to while simultaneously having to complete the full-time job of skillfully filleting her independent self from the body of her family. This was, to my way of thinking, the main reason she had begun smoking pot so regularly—getting high was the only way she had found to unburden herself, even temporarily, from the encumbrance of these unattainable objectives.

It is essential that parents find ways to view their children's problems as attempts to *solve* a problem. In so doing, they not only are able to be more empathic and understanding but can then help their children to find a better, more adaptive solution to the problem they have (often unwittingly) been trying to solve.

Once Amanda's parents began to realize that her problem behaviors were the result of her trying to address the unresolved problems embedded in her family's history, they were able to start addressing and resolving these problems themselves. This shift in their outlook automatically changed, in positive ways, how they saw Amanda, which in turn automatically changed, in positive ways, how she saw herself. So, as I helped them to see *through* her, they were better able to see her through.

Along these lines, one particularly heartwarming turning point in treatment occurred when I asked Amanda and her father to spend an afternoon together, first visiting Aunt Delia's grave site (which Amanda had never been to) and then visiting the grave site of her friend Daryl, the one who had been killed in a car accident. Amanda told me during a subsequent session that it was "the first time I ever really saw my father cry and probably the first time in a long time that I let him see *me* cry." Helping them both to mourn, and to connect with each other *around* their mourning, freed Amanda from having to constantly work overtime to speak to the grief that had remained, for so long, unspoken. And what is unspoken in families eventually becomes unspeakable.

As I also mentioned in the epilogue, Amanda's parents were eventually willing, with my encouragement, to take a closer look at their marriage and to join with me to find ways to resuscitate and reinvigorate their relationship with each other. This, too, seemed to give the family a good deal of therapeutic thrust and traction and rock all of them out of their rut; as they worked to untie some long-standing relational knots, they were then free to move closer to each other in new and more appropriate ways.

Involved, open-minded parents will usually find that they get as much from their children as they give, sometimes even more. Our children's issues always force us to examine our own, and in that sense, parenthood can help to grow *us* up, which in turn makes it more likely that our children will grow up too.

Regarding the issue of parent-teen communication, many of the parents who come to me complaining that they can't communicate with their teen seem to have too narrowly defined the nature of communication. Communication to them means "My son happily gushes forth with everything that is going on in his life" or "My daughter agrees with what I say and does what I tell her to." While the topic of parent-teen communication is worthy of a book all its own rather than just a few paragraphs, I have found in general that there are two simple rules when it comes to establishing adequate communication with teens—adolescents will not speak if they don't feel that they're going to be listened to, and they will not listen if we don't speak to them with candor, care, and respect.

This may come as a surprise to you, but all the adolescents that I've worked with truly *want* to be able to communicate more effectively with their parents, want to listen and to be heard, to understand and to be understood, but they haven't always been able to find a way to do so that doesn't threaten to crush in some way the fragile eggshell of their identity.

Amanda helped me to see right away that having a weekly face-to-face conversation with her was out of the question. But that left me to reflect upon a related question—"If we're not going to talk, how else might we connect?" Parents should never underestimate the power of words, but sometimes you have to find the right vehicle to carry those words. If it's not a spoken transaction, then it can be a letter or an e-mail or an exchange of instant messages.

I have witnessed many teens turning their backs on and closing their minds to a long-winded lecture from their mother or father, but most adolescents' inquisitiveness will be aroused by, for example, discovering an envelope with their name on it taped to their bedroom door and will subsequently feel compelled to open it and read the letter inside (even if they refrain from acknowledging that they ever did so or from responding to it). Don't ever assume that an absence of communication with your teen suggests a lack of interest in communication—it's usually just a matter of establishing the right communicative apparatus.

Finally, it was crucial for me to find a way to maneuver Amanda's parents through the treacherous shoals of unnecessary guilt. As I noted above, blame of self or others plays no salutary role when it comes to effective parenting. There are no perfect parents, nor is it necessary that we ever feel compelled to *be* perfect parents, and none of us gets through child rearing without experiencing lacerating remorse and searing regret regarding what we said or didn't say, did or didn't do. I like to joke with parents that if we *were* perfect, the unfavorable outcome would be that our children would never want to leave us. And of course, our children wouldn't learn to gracefully accept their own imperfections unless we were constantly modeling our own imperfections, plus some grudging self-acceptance for them.

Our job as mothers and fathers is not to always try to do things the "right way" (as if there actually *were* a right way) but just to have more faith in our children than they have in themselves; to become a beacon that guides their way forward and a mirror that reflects back to them the image of them at their finest; and to deal, with as much balance and optimism as possible, with family life's inevitable gusts and squalls, swirls and eddies, unafraid to share the love, care, and hope that bind us to each other and that lead us all to more humane ways of being in the world.

Amanda's parents deserve tremendous credit for hanging in there with her through a frightening and formidable time, for persisting in the face of tremendous despair and disappointment, for being willing to allow themselves to evolve, and for never letting go of the redemptive possibilities of family love.

———

We are poor indeed if we are only sane.

−D. W. WINNICOTT

You are lost the instant you know
what the result will be.

−JUAN GRIS

A NOTE TO PROFESSIONALS

Psychological treatment should unfold so much more smoothly and work so much more efficiently than it ever really does. After all, the patient wants to change and get better, and the clinician has the skills and the desire to help him or her to do so—why, then, does it have to get so bewildering and byzantine?

In this final section, which is geared mostly toward psychotherapists but which will also be of use to educators, adolescent medicine specialists, health care providers, clergy, and other professionals who guide and care for teenagers, I will briefly discuss the therapeutic relationship that evolved between Amanda and me and use it as a way to explore the kaleidoscopic complexity of healing adolescent anguish.

When I first met with Amanda and her parents, it became clear to me that my initial and most important clinical task was to woo them out of the quagmire that they had become stuck in, the one built upon the immobilizing premise that Amanda was damaged and deficient and that there was little her parents could do to help, since her difficulties were the inevitable result of deep-rooted, individually based psychopathology.

As I told Amanda in one of my first letters, we have done families a great disservice by so rigidly defining what health and sanity are and by characterizing even the tiniest departures from this highly restricted norm as signs of emotional disturbance and mental illness. By taking a therapeutic ax to the frozen sea of this family's assumptions, contaminating the trancelike perspective they had adopted, and inviting them all, Amanda included, to look differently at who she was and why she behaved the way she did, I may have made them a little more permeable to change, which initiated the process of getting them unstuck.

I have become convinced through my years of practice that psychological symptoms can best be understood not as a failure of the individual but as a failure of the imagination, an inability, as I mentioned in the preceding note to parents, to conceptualize and articulate problematic behavior as essentially health-based and problem *solving*. The more hospitality we can display toward the incomplete, missing, contradictory, and paradoxical parts of ourselves; the more mercy we can dispense in response to our stubborn flaws and weaknesses; and the more we can love ourselves *because* of, rather than in spite of, our limitations and liabilities, then the greater the likelihood that we can transcend and transform our "symptoms" and travel from the land of "There must be something wrong with me" to the land of "There must be something important that I am trying to say."

It was also necessary for me to not too meagerly specify and stipulate what the enterprise of psychotherapy consisted of. Just because Amanda didn't feel optimistic or trusting enough to verbally open up her heart to me right away didn't mean that her painful silence wasn't hurting her. It was up to me to find an innovative way *into* her silence and to help decode and soften it, rather than to intractably insist that we proceed in complete compliance with the traditional rituals of treatment—coming in, sitting down, talking for fifty minutes, and then leaving. That may work for some adolescents (or at least be tolerated by some), but I seriously doubt that it works for most.

At times these letters seemed to me to function like a fragile string between the tin cans of our respective hearts, slowly transporting back and forth the substance of what we wanted to convey to each other. At other times the exchange of our letters felt like a form of human echolocation, each of us cautiously broadcasting our pulsed signals and anxiously awaiting the reverberation in a gradual and persistent effort to find ourselves and each other.

It was by design, in fact, that I chose to use snail mail rather than e-mail to write to Amanda, because I felt that making this very delicate process more concrete (a letter in hand) and less instantaneous (taking a couple of days rather than a couple of seconds) would give it additional force and urgency. That she responded in kind suggests that she felt the same way.

Keeping the focus on Amanda's intrinsic strengths and abilities was, in retrospect, indispensable as well. Adolescents already feel inadequate and insufficient enough without having a therapist stride gallantly onto the scene to *fix* them, to confiscate their hard-earned identities and dictate to them what they must do in order to change and be cured. The more responsible we feel ourselves to be for teens' growth, the less likely they are to actually grow—we must aim for *responsiveness* more than responsibility.

And although we may indeed be the experts and the authorities on psychological development *in general,* we have to convey to our patients that they are the experts and authorities on *themselves.* Amanda actually told me during one of our final sessions, when we were discussing what I had done that had and had not been helpful to her, that I was the first clinician who appeared more interested in *knowing* her than in helping her or making her "better."

In successful treatment it is not so much that the therapist *provides* relief, resolution, and healing as that his or her empathic presence, thought-provoking questions, and novel frameworks serve to attract the patient's curiosity and provide her with the space, the strategies, and the motivation to *find* relief, resolution, and healing. The therapist becomes the midwife to the birth of the adolescent's embryonic adult identity, the provisional custodian of her forsaken health and potential until she is able to claim, trust, and embody them herself.

While the relationship that I developed with Amanda through our letter writing was an individual one that, by definition, excluded her parents, I am sure that it is abundantly clear to readers that her treatment was still family based. The letters were never designed to be a therapeutic end point but instead were envisioned as a starting point in building the foundation for the conjoint work that would ultimately be necessary to promote enduring change in the family system.

As Amanda's confidence in our collaboration grew through the exchange of letters, I was eventually able to establish more traditional family therapy sessions as our most salient clinical modality, and everyone, as we have seen, reaped the benefits.

Whenever there are family matters to attend to, the more that the entire family is participating, the more progress is likely to be made, and the sturdier that progress is likely to be. Discussion and disclosure are ultimately useless exercises unless they are translated into action, and the most therapeutic action will take place when the family has the chance to unite and reconfigure their stifling patterns of interaction in vivo, as a group. An investment in one well-constructed family session will always pay off more handsomely than dozens of teen-opening-up-to-her-therapist-about-her-mean-parents or parents-lamenting-their-whiny-selfish-teen appointments.

Ultimately, though, it's a matter of therapeutic outlook rather than who is or is not sitting in the consultation room. For example, I have supervised clinicians who have invited numerous family members into their office for sessions but who are still misled into thinking that the problems of the identified patient exist within him or her rather than within the confounding web of family relationships. And I have supervised others who literally see only one patient in their office but who bring a systemic, family-based orientation to their work with that patient.

There *were* some clinical risks that I had to consider as I launched and undertook an in-depth, between-sessions correspondence with Amanda, however. I needed to constantly regulate my tendency to side with "poor Amanda" against her sometimes stoic, inflexible parents when it came to rules and restrictions and at the same time reinforce their authority and the parental hierarchy without completely antagonizing her, a delicate balance that was not always possible to sustain.

And I had to monitor my desire to compete successfully with Amanda's father and conscientiously attempt to outdo him as the main paternal figure in her life. This would have been gratifying for *me,* in some ways, but it would ultimately have worked against Amanda's development, as she already had a competent father whom she needed to work things out with, and she would be maintaining a lifetime relationship with *him,* not me.

On the other hand, I did hope, and had some reason to believe, that my epistolary alliance with Amanda would provide him with a template for how a father could commence a dialogue with an adolescent daughter and would maybe even agitate some dormant rivalry with me that would spur him to overcome his isolation and invite her back into closer contact.

In any case, framing my one-to-one relationship with Amanda as a bridge that would move the entire family closer to each other and to health and resilience, which was understood by both her and her parents, seems to have worked decently enough.

Because the reader has been exposed only to my letters to Amanda and not hers to me, it should certainly not be inferred that she was always happy with me and my approach. There were plenty of times, initially conveyed to me in her letters (such as chapter 12, "How *Dare* You") and later on directly during sessions, when she complained bitterly about my insensitivity, when she irritably blew off my well-meant theories and hypotheses, and when she became irate with me when she felt that I was aligning with her parents against her.

To me, however, as I discussed with Amanda, these were sure signs that a real therapeutic relationship was developing. Therapists cannot *help* but annoy, disappoint, neglect, and injure their patients, just as parents cannot help doing the same with their children—it is built into our role, and if it's not happening at all, chances are that we're not taking our role seriously enough. But minor and major breaks in empathy, affection, and connectedness between therapist and patient (and also between parent and adolescent), troubling as they may be, are absolutely vital and hold forth great healing properties if embraced and explored. When these relational ruptures occurred, Amanda had to see that I could handle her feelings of rage, violation, and betrayal without my collapsing or retaliating, that I could remain interested in her and caring toward her even if she wasn't going to submerge these feelings in another self-sacrificial effort to be a "good girl."

I have learned the hard way that therapy is most therapeutic when the therapist is somehow able to tolerate and identify with, rather than ignore and negate, the patient's feelings of anger and futility, anger and futility that naturally spur the same discomfiting emotions within us. In several of her letters, Amanda wondered, "Why haven't you given up on me yet?" and, to be truthful, there were certainly times when I was feeling just as trounced as she was, when it seemed that we'd all be better off if I would simply capitulate, wearily write her off as just another lost cause, pigeonhole her neatly in some diagnostic category, and renounce trying to infuse this hopeless situation with any hope. Therapy always takes place at the intersection of doubt and belief, and it's not always clear which avenue is going to be traveled.

But it was also clear that Amanda needed me to play the role of something like a "psychological dialysis unit," shunting over to me all of her most dangerous emotionality so that I could temporarily house, process, and purify it and then return it to her without its feeling so worrisome and hazardous. It seemed extremely important for her that I understand with lapidary precision and correctness her sense of the impossibility of it all and to share the experience of that impossibility with her so that she was no longer alone with it.

All of us, during our bleakest times, are looking for some kind of containment for our most dreadful feelings, and while sometimes chemical (psychotropic medicine) and/or institutional (clinics, hospitals, detention centers, prisons) containment become warranted, as they had been for a time in Amanda's case, it is usually a strong, capacious, interpersonal containment that we seek and that holds forth the most profound healing powers. No matter how much we eventually learn about human genetics and physiology, there will never be a clinical substitute for the deeply human need to be compassionately heard, held, and understood, in whatever form these encounters can best take place.

Because the reader has also not been exposed to the content of my sessions with Amanda's parents, it should not be assumed that they always concurred with my theories and hypotheses either. Her mother and father entered my office quite stonily and skeptically (understandably, based on their difficult life histories and their previous experiences with therapeutic futility), giving me very little to work with. And there was initially a very reassuring (albeit debilitating) sense of helplessness that they hugged around themselves—reassuring because it excused them from any responsibility for the current state of affairs—one that they fought long and hard to maintain despite my most concerted efforts to deprogram them. Just as I was tempted, at times, to write Amanda off out of frustration and fatigue, I was tempted at times to write her remote parents off as well.

But it always helped to keep in the front of my mind how much sorrow these two individuals had had to endure in their lives. After all, it wasn't just Amanda but her mother and father as well who needed me—to make sense of their fears; to bear witness to their deep-seated grief; to yoke together the scattered, shattered nuclei of their collective self-worth; to reteach to them the lessons of love that had weakened in the thickets of their tremendous losses; to be near and present as they took a deep breath, stared down over their steep emotional cliffs, and perhaps for the first time ever, bravely contemplated the fearsome landscapes that loomed below.

One final challenge that it feels important to acknowledge was having to come to grips with the limits of my influence over Amanda. I have always believed that we make of therapy not what we wish but what we can. As discussed in the epilogue, while she improved in many ways, I wasn't able to talk Amanda out of a reliance on pot and alcohol or her at times promiscuous sexual behavior (although she did eventually relinquish both). Despite repeated efforts during the course of our work together, I could never persuade her to adopt a regular exercise regime or begin the day with a nourishing breakfast or practice meditation.

But coming to terms with the limits of empathy and compassion, and of experience and expertise, is a necessary step in treatment because it reminds us, and our patients, that we do not maintain sovereignty over them, that they are ultimately free agents who make their own choices. Frustrating as this may be to recognize, particularly when we believe we "know what's best" for a patient, it is also liberating for both of us. This is especially true for the adolescent patient, whose main objective is to extricate and emancipate herself from the dominion of others and stake out an independent empire of her own. We must all realize that the key to life's engine is always found *inside* oneself, not outside.

On a concluding note, therapy, as I proposed in the epilogue, should not extend forever but should have "term limits"—it works best not as an open-ended process but as one that puts us in the position of being better able to endure and survive life's inevitable cruelties and absurdities, its dizzying cycles of triumph and defeat, fulfillment and emptiness, enlightenment and disillusionment, by utilizing our own resources and relationships. I knew from the very moment that we started treatment, as I do with all of my patients, that

Amanda and I would have to finish treatment, and just as an awareness of mortality sharpens our desire to live our lives more fully, an awareness of the finality of treatment sharpens our desire to accomplish what needs to be accomplished so that the patient (and therapist) can proceed forward.

It was necessary for Amanda to be able to idealize me, to treasure and cherish what I had given her during the time that we worked together, but it was unquestionably just as important for her to leave me behind and begin to see that she could do without me. Only then could we both know that the treatment that we worked so hard at had ultimately been as successful and rewarding as we hoped it would be.

———

And the song goes on, beautiful.

—RAINER MARIA RILKE

—

ACKNOWLEDGMENTS

While this book is, in some ways, a distillation of all that I have learned about psychotherapy and human development from countless colleagues, supervisors, teachers, and authors over the years, my in-depth consultations, collaborations, and/or conversations with the following clinicians at various points in my professional journey have been particularly instrumental and influential when it came to the development of my approach to treatment, and to them I offer my heartfelt gratitude.

HALCY BOHEN, PHD
THOMAS BURNS, PHD
GEORGE COHEN, MA
RUTH LEBOVITZ, DSW
ROGER LEWIN, MD

Elena Manzanera, ms

Karen Meckler, md

Phyllis Stern, ma

Ellen Talles, lcsw, adtr

Jill Woleslagle, lcsw–c

Thanks also to my still-adamantine agent, Sarah Jane Freymann, for her interest in and support of my work over the years, and for her unhesitating willingness to separate the literary wheat from the chaff; and to my editor, Eden Steinberg, for her faith in these letters and her willingness to broadcast the message that they yearn to carry.

A portion of the profits from the sale of this book will be donated by the author to Grassroots Crisis Intervention Center in Columbia, Maryland, and to the Neurotrauma Unit of Johns Hopkins University Hospital in Baltimore, Maryland.

ABOUT THE AUTHOR

Dr. Brad Sachs is a family psychologist and the author, most recently, of *The Good Enough Child* and *The Good Enough Teen*. He completed his undergraduate work at Brown University, and his doctorate at University of Maryland, College Park.

A former secondary schoolteacher, he is also the founder and director of The Father Center, a program designed to meet the needs of new, expectant, and experienced fathers.

Dr. Sachs is nationally renowned for his creative and innovative treatment of families, and his workshops and seminars. He has contributed articles to numerous popular and professional journals, travels and lectures frequently, and is a regular guest on radio and television talk shows. He has explored the kaleidoscopic complexity of family life not only in his clinical work and writings, but also through poetry and music.

Dr. Sachs is married to Dr. Karen Meckler, a psychiatrist and medical acupuncturist. Together they raise their three teenaged children, Josh, Matt, and Jessica, and their two dogs in Columbia, Maryland.

He can be contacted directly through his web site: www.bradsachs.com.

BRADSACHS.COM

Visit *www.bradsachs.com* to download discussion guides designed specifically for teens, for parents, or for professionals (including educators, clergy, mental health professionals, and others who work with adolescents). These guides can be used in a variety of contexts including:

- Book clubs for teens and/or parents
- Youth groups
- PTA and community meetings
- Faculty in-service workshops
- Inpatient and outpatient support and therapy groups for adolescents
- High school and college psychology classes

- Enhancing individual experience and perspective while reading *When No One Understands*

Dr. Sachs also welcomes letters from readers, which he'll respond to as time allows. Letters can be e-mailed to him through his website or sent to the following mailing address:

Dr. Brad Sachs
Suite 3
Stevens Forest Professional Center
9650 Santiago Road
Columbia, MD 21045